THE
NEW MOTHER'S BODY BOOK

JACQUELINE SHANNON

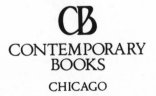

CONTEMPORARY
BOOKS

CHICAGO

Library of Congress Cataloging-in-Publication Data

Shannon, Jacqueline.
    The new mother's body book / Jacqueline Shannon.
       p.   cm.
    Includes index.
    ISBN 0-8092-3795-4
    1. Posnatal care.   2. Puerperium.   3. Mothers—
Health and hygiene.   I. Title.
RG801.S45   1994
618.6—dc20   93-46066
                                    CIP

Published by Contemporary Books, Inc.
Two Prudential Plaza, Chicago, Illinois 60601-6790
Manufactured in the United States of America
International Standard Book Number: 0-8092-3795-4
10   9   8   7   6   5   4   3   2   1

For Catherine Nicholas Cento,
who has been there for me
during all of my "pod person" periods
(including the year after Madeline's birth)

CONTENTS

PART ONE: BODY

PART TWO: SOUL

PREGNANCY CHANGES YOU FOREVER

Not long ago, I was in the pregnancy and childbirth section of a local bookstore where I found hundreds of books on breastfeeding, baby care, and parenting in general. But nowhere did I see a book like *The New Mother's Body Book*, a book specifically devoted to what happens to Mom after the baby is born. Sure, you might run across a few pages dealing with episiotomies and engorged breasts in one book and a quick "how to resume sexual relations" in another. But this kind of in-depth study of the physical and emotional changes that a woman experiences—not only in the immediate postpartum period but in the months and years thereafter—is unique. Even the obstetrics textbook in my office fails to offer this kind of insight.

As a physician who has practiced obstetrics and gynecology for ten years, I initially sat down to read *The New Mother's Body Book* primarily to ensure that it contained no medical misinformation. Of course I found the facts to be current and reliable. But as I read along, my reactions became less and less intellectual and more and more emotional and maternal. Jacqueline Shannon puts into words information that is universal to motherhood. There are pearls that my professors didn't teach me in medical school, that my mother didn't tell me, and that my best friends and I never discussed. As the mother of two young children, I realized that this was a book needed in the postpartum months as much as Dr. Spock.

At one point, I found myself remembering how, shortly after I gave birth to my first baby, I set a goal that I'd be able to wear a clingy St. John knit (a bikini never even made it on my list!) within six months. Well, my daughter is now eight years old, and I still haven't ventured into the St. John section of my favorite department store, nor would I even if there was a big SALE! sign hung over it. You see, I have run, stepped, lifted weights, and stretched in gyms all over town, but the inches that were once part of my breasts are now firmly attached to my waist. Until now, no source has so concisely and candidly informed women that this can happen—and furthermore that it is *common*. Nor had I ever dreamed, before I had my children, that motherhood would not only change the way I deal with problems on a daily basis but also my perception of the world and even of my community (I left a busy practice in one city and started all over in another just to put my kids in a better school system!).

In today's society, many women survive the stresses of parenthood without the support of an extended family of "wise women" for shared experiences and support. Groups such as Lamaze and La Leche League fill some of these gaps. But these groups focus on the woman as she is important to the child, not on the woman herself. The fact is that a woman who has had a baby has undergone a tremendous physical, emotional, and hormonal ordeal, usually without much help. *The New Mother's Body Book* focuses solely on the woman and what happens to her body and her mind after she has had her child; it helps remind her that although there is now a new, all-consuming little person who is needy twenty-four hours a day, she and her marriage are also deserving of time and attention.

Jacqueline Shannon has compiled an amazing amount of practical information and advice for new mothers in this easy-to-read volume. Sometimes you'll find yourself laughing as you read; other times, you'll gasp, "That's me!"

There is much for everyone in *The New Mother's Body Book.* If you're planning to get pregnant for the first time (or are in the midst of your first pregnancy), you'll find it brimming with news, support, and suggestions. If you're a mother planning a second pregnancy, you'll find plenty of valuable information just for you. And anyone in the health care field who works with pregnant or new mothers will find this book indispensable. As someone who has been in all three positions, I highly recommend it.

Neysa Whiteman, M.D., mother of two, is board-certified in obstetrics and gynecology. She practices in San Diego, California.

MANY THANKS

. . . to my friend Stacy Prince, who had so much enthusiasm about this book and so much conviction that it was needed and whose insights and leads were invaluable (and who—incidentally—was my editor!).

. . . to Julie Castiglia for her powers of persuasion.

. . . to my sisters, Sally Jones and Barbara Richards, and my friends Rachel McCurry and Roberta Lorbeer for relating their experiences; and also to all of my friends who were generous with their input but not with the use of their real names!

. . . to the many doctors and others who shared their expertise—particularly Neysa Whiteman, Sheryl Cramer, Leslie Mark, Deborah Nemiro, John Winder, Doris Flood, Carol Ann Weber, and Sheila Cluff—and who didn't grow exasperated when I continually pressed "But is that *permanent?*"

. . . to my husband, Stephen Trobaugh, and my daughter, Madeline, who have graciously allowed me to use them in so many anecdotes and who patiently and politely tried to ignore my side of phone conversations about such things as fat cells and hemorrhoids—sometimes over meals!—during the research phase.

. . . and to all of the women who sat next to me on airplanes or stood behind me in supermarket lines and shared intimate details about their postpartum selves but whose names I neglected to get.

INTRODUCTION

In the first two years after my daughter, Madeline, was born, I interviewed fifty or more mothers of young children—formally, for various parenting articles, and informally, when Madeline and I would do the local playground or birthday party. Combining the input of these mothers with my own experience, I discovered Three Great Truths:

1. After nine months of being coddled, coached, and clucked over by doctors, nurses, Lamaze instructors, family, pregnancy books, and grandmotherly strangers at the mall, a new mother is virtually abandoned once the standard six-week postpartum period has passed, even though . . .
2. She has almost certainly not "snapped out of it" either physically or mentally, and . . .
3. Nobody ever told her that many of the changes pregnancy wrought on her body would be permanent! To her surprise, she learns that once you have a baby, you have a different body forever.

The seeds for Great Truth Number 1 were sown when a friend asked me if it was considered abnormal for sex to still be uncomfortable seven months after birth. Her doctor, who had examined her reproductive organs six weeks after birth and then again some months later after a pap smear, had pronounced her "fit as a fiddle" each time, and she was too embarrassed to ask the sex question. "There is an immense gap between fiddle and diddle, and I could not bridge that," she explained to me with a wry smile.

I went in search of a book or magazine article to help her. And came up with zip. The few books dealing specifically with the postpartum period—and the magazine articles and chapters in pregnancy-and-birth books devoted to this subject—generally cover just the first six or eight weeks after birth, and/or they gloss over the mother's adjustments in favor of the baby's.

Weeks passed, and more moms (via phone interviews and in the park) adamantly confirmed my growing suspicion that crystallized into Great Truth Number 2: the postpartum period lasts much longer for most women than just a couple of months. Then bits and pieces from "official" sources drifted in to back that up. I came across a study at the University of Pennsylvania School of Nursing, for example, that found that almost half of seventy women surveyed hadn't regained their usual energy two months after childbirth. I also heard about a "postpartum" support group a psychologist in Berkeley, California, had formed specifically to help women who were unhappy with their after-baby bodies. Most of the mothers who joined were far from being new mothers. Some had given birth six years earlier! Additional research in the bookstore led me to conclude that not only is there a dearth of information about postpartum adjustments after the first few weeks, much of the after-baby advice for new mothers is overly—

almost cruelly—optimistic. You're led to believe that there's something weird or sluggish or just plain wrong with you if you aren't back to normal in two months. Several books, for example, assure new moms that with "a little work" they'll have their old waistlines back within two months. Ha!

Great Truth Number 3 had its roots in the birthday party of a little girl who turned two the same summer Madeline did. A bunch of us fairly new mothers were sitting around watching the kids smash cake into the patio bricks when Amy, the birthday girl's mom, bragged that she hadn't had a single menstrual cramp since her daughter was born. This woman used to suffer such agonizing pains that she would practically OD on ibuprofen every month.

The rest of us were eager to throw in our own postpregnancy body differences, and unfortunately not all of them were so wonderful. "I think pregnancy rearranged my insides so that my bladder is much smaller than it used to be," said my friend Gail, for example. "I have to get up twice a night to go to the bathroom." Lora, who had an eleven-month-old, shook her head sadly. "My doctor says he doesn't care if I do eighteen hundred sit-ups a day," she said. "He says once you have a baby your stomach will never be as flat as it was before." As for me, I reported that shortly after delivering my daughter almost two years earlier, the number of migraine headaches I suffer in a month increased significantly. I also developed hay fever. Gina, who had her second baby a week after I had my first, complained that since the birth of her children she gets a backache any time she stands in one place longer than five minutes. Finally, five of the six of us declared that our breasts are smaller than they were prepregnancy . . . as much as one cup size, in one case.

This discussion really got us thinking. Many of us knew well in advance about the changes to expect in the immediate postpartum period—the shrinking of the uterus and so forth. But nobody—not our obstetricians, our Lamaze instructors, our pregnancy-and-birth books, or our mothers—ever told us that pregnancy has such a radical effect on the body that it can make permanent changes. But can it? Or were the positives and negatives we listed that day purely coincidental in their timing or just part of the natural aging process?

I snared a magazine assignment to find out, and my first surprise was how hard it was to get the answers. It seemed to me that there was almost a conspiracy out there to keep the information I sought secret lest women would decide to forego babymaking for the sake of their bodies. I ended up having to divide the postpregnancy body into parts and to consult a variety of specialists, such as a dermatologist, a plastic surgeon, and a physician who specializes in premenstrual syndrome (PMS). In the course of explaining the aftereffects of pregnancy on particular parts of the body, all the specialists reported that mothers with postpregnancy-related complaints were common in their practices.

The host of permanent "souvenirs" of pregnancy that I learned about—souvenirs that can occur literally from head to toe—astonished me, a writer who had specialized in women's health issues for ten years. Once you have a baby, you truly do have a different body forever. I learned, for example, about a fact of life called postpartum atrophy, a condition that leaves the breasts forever smaller after birth than they were prepregnancy and that affects 90 percent of all women who have given birth. (The plastic surgeon I asked to explain this process told me that 50 percent of his breast augmentation patients seek the surgery because of postpartum atrophy.) I learned that lots of women have a permanent reduction in bladder capacity. I also learned that I wasn't the only woman who had to buy larger shoes after having a child.

This all sounds pretty depressing, doesn't it? I thought so, too. In fact, when I decided to pitch the idea of writing a book that would cover not just this subject (to my frustration, my magazine article barely touched on the basics, thanks to space restrictions) but would address Great Truths 1 and 2 as well, I gave it a depressing title: *Beyond Stretch Marks.*

Then something extraordinary happened. My thinking began to turn around on this subject. Part of the reason for this was strictly personal. As Madeline grew older, my life became less frantic. I had more time to devote to myself (enough time, for example, to get a really good, flattering haircut instead of just the hurried bang trim I used to be relegated to with a toddler bouncing on my lap). I got more sleep. I had more time to exercise. My confidence in my looks began to return. I stopped getting every single cold or flu bug that Madeline brought home from preschool. About the time she turned four, I found myself thinking that physically I felt as good as I ever had. And then came this astonishing topper: One night, as I was getting undressed for bed, my husband, Steve, looked at me and remarked, "You know, you have a better butt than you had before Madeline."

My change of heart continued as I delved into medical research and interviewed more mothers for this book. I heard about Olympic runners whose pregnancies *improved* their times. I discovered that pregnancy and childbirth often cure women of endometriosis (the presence of uterine lining tissue outside the uterus) and chronic fatigue syndrome, that giving birth not only reduces your chances of getting breast and other female cancers but also signifi-

cantly decreases your risk of contracting seemingly nonre-
lated cancers, such as *brain* cancer. I talked to lots of
women who are thrilled that motherhood has increased
their confidence in themselves, and to others who have
gained a whole new appreciation for our gender and who
find that their relationships with their mothers and girl-
friends are now deeper and richer. I interviewed women
who were amazed at the endurance motherhood bestows
on a woman and at how they can nurse a sick child for
most of the night and still show up at work on time the
next morning, while a similarly sleep-deprived night of
cramming in college necessitated a week of recuperation. I
met women who feel much more a part of their community—and who have gained a whole new reverence and
concern for our *world*—since they crossed the great divide
into motherhood.

What is the difference between most of *these* women
and all those grousing women at the long-ago birthday
party? Like me, they have been mothers for at least three
years. They have gotten past those frantic first two, when
your world seemingly shrinks to just you and your baby
and your body is still trying to recover from the enormous
upheaval of pregnancy and childbirth.

The upshot of all this is that, while I still believe in all
three of my Great Truths and have written this book to
rectify them, I have revised my thinking on Great Truth 3.
Sure, a lot of the changes wrought by pregnancy and
childbirth are permanent, but they're not all bad. In fact,
I truly believe that if you hang in there for a couple of
years, you come out—on balance—not just new but
improved.

Not that I have whitewashed things here. Despite my
overall change of heart, you'll find the negative souvenirs
of pregnancy—the varicose veins, the stress incontinence,

the PMS—described in glorious detail. I also cover the mental drawbacks of motherhood—the stress, the anxiety. But this book is packed with good news, too. If you are suffering a bout of morning sickness as you read these pages, are queasily questioning whether getting pregnant was such a good idea after all, nervously wondering, "What have I gotten myself into?," by the time you finish this book, I think your answer will be "Something wonderful."

Jaqueline Shannon

PART ONE:
BODY

CHAPTER ONE

THE FIRST SIX WEEKS

Initial Transitions

The premise of this book is that motherhood turns you into a different person both physically and mentally . . . and that if you add up all the minuses, you come out not just different but *better*. You are not going to see it that way in the first six weeks, however.

At no other time in your life will your body and your mind experience the same amount of upheaval that occurs in the first several weeks after your baby is born. I read in a medical journal, for example, that if you were to lose as much weight at any other time in your life as fast as you do in the first week after childbirth, your body would go into shock. All that your systems took nine leisurely months to do, they race to undo—in order to prepare you as quickly as possible to go through the whole thing again, should you desire to. You will also wrestle with conflicting and sometimes strange or even troubling emotions, some of them hormonally bred and some not. All of this will be exacerbated by fatigue—first as a result of labor and delivery

(Sheldon H. Cherry, an obstetrician/gynecologist, once wrote that you expend as much energy giving birth as you would by hiking twelve miles) and then because of the unrelenting, sleep-depriving demands of a newborn. That these parenting tasks are not only unrelenting but unfamiliar, even scary, adds to the stress. "I went into pregnancy a highly competent, completely confident woman who was a whiz at reading profit and loss statements and even fixing my car," said my friend Darcie. "And there I stood six days after my baby's birth, supposedly still the same woman but frozen with fear, over her bottom, thermometer in hand, for at least five minutes. The pediatrician had instructed me over the phone to take her temperature rectally, and I was terrified that I would stick it in wrong and hurt her."

One final reason why the first six weeks are especially tough is that the medical community pretty much abandons the new mother. Most of the women I interviewed for this book felt they got great postpartum care while they were in the hospital. "In fact," said my friend Glenda, "when they're coming around every few hours to take your temperature and massage your uterus, you get to the point where you wish they'd leave you alone so you can get some sleep, for crying out loud. But once it's time to leave, they pack you up, they thrust a few booklets into your hands, and the attitude becomes 'You're on your own, Mom.'"

"All of the focus suddenly shifts from you to your baby," another mom said. "And that's true not just of doctors and nurses but of most of the 'having a baby' books out there, as well. They jump right from the labor and delivery chapter to the one about taking care of your new baby."

Some people in the medical community *are* beginning to address this neglect. In early 1993, Dwenda K. Gjerdingen, M.D., of the School of Public Health at the University of Minnesota released a landmark study done in 1989 of

436 first-time mothers in St. Paul and their physical health during the year after they gave birth. Summarizing her study in a medical journal, Gjerdingen began by saying that recovery from childbirth is often viewed by the medical community "as a relatively uneventful course that requires little assistance from health care providers, as demonstrated by the single postpartum visit typically recommended several weeks after delivery." Additional contacts with nurses or physicians during this period are usually for the purpose of monitoring the infant's rather than the mother's well-being, Gjerdingen said, but she added that "a closer look at the postpartum period reveals that, for many women, recovery from childbirth is not always so simple. The majority of women probably contend with several minor to moderate discomforts for weeks, and some face more serious problems that may limit important daily functions for some time."

My own most memorable postpartum experience with the medical community occurred several weeks after I delivered my daughter, Madeline. I called the large HMO I belong to and asked for an appointment with the wonderful nurse-midwife who had attended the birth. I explained to the receptionist that I was having problems with my episiotomy. "She only sees pregnant women," was the receptionist's curt reply. She wouldn't even let me talk to the midwife by phone. When I told another new mother this story recently, she nodded her head in empathy and said, "It's like suddenly being kicked out of a club that all of your best friends still belong to."

Because I remember that keen sense of abandonment so well, I decided this book should include detailed information about those first few transitional weeks as well as the long-term and permanent changes having a baby makes. In this chapter, we'll cover the physical transitions to expect after you leave the hospital; Chapter 3 has suggestions for coping with these conditions; and in Chapter 7, in the "Soul" part of this book, you'll find information about the emotional highs and lows that are common in the first few weeks of motherhood.

Physical Transitions in the First Six Weeks

Your uterus will continue to contract. In the first six postpartum weeks, thanks to a process called involution, the uterus shrinks twentyfold—from about two pounds to two ounces—and returns to a lower position in the pelvic cavity. Already, by the end of labor, its upper edge is below the belly button. If you feel your uterus right after delivery, after the placenta and amniotic fluid have been expelled, you'll find it's about the size of a grapefruit. Within two weeks, you'll have trouble locating it.

To accomplish this shrinkage, as well as to expel any blood or pieces of placenta that remain, the uterus contracts. These contractions are called *afterpains.* Each usually lasts less than a minute; they can continue for two or three days after birth (although I talked to one woman who had them for a month). If you had a relatively painless, medicated birth, afterpains might seem surprisingly strong. But because my labor was unmedicated, I considered my afterpains a relative picnic—no worse than menstrual cramps, and afterpains aren't continuous like menstrual cramps are. Apparently, however, afterpains are much more painful after a second or subsequent birth (see Chapter 6).

Breastfeeding speeds up involution because the baby's sucking releases a hormone called oxytocin that stimulates uterine contractions. It is common for new mothers to feel afterpains at the start of early nursing sessions.

You will have a bloody discharge. Officially known as *lochia,* your postpartum discharge consists of blood from the site where the placenta detached, any remaining bits of placenta, and the lining of the uterus. This discharge starts out to be very heavy and bright red, changes to brown in a week or two (an indication that no new bleeding is occurring), then turns yellowish or even clear. While researching this process, I came across some experts who wrote that women who had C-sections and women who breastfeed have a lighter lochia flow. But I asked women who'd had both vaginal and cesarean births if they noticed any difference in the lochia between the two births; they hadn't. And I am at least one breastfeeding mother who had a very heavy flow. The average amount of lochia expelled is supposedly—and surprisingly—only one pint, and three-quarters of that amount is expelled in the first four days after birth.

The entire process takes about three to six weeks, and to cope with it you'll need a supply of large sanitary pads. It's feared that wearing tampons during the first week or two after birth, while the cervix is still so open, might promote a uterine infection. (And if you had an episiotomy, you won't feel like using tampons for a while anyway.) Don't balk at the industrial-sized pads the hospital supplies. You may feel as though you're wearing a saddle, but you *need* a saddle, especially in the first few days, when it seems like you're constantly needing to change pads.

Incidentally, a lot of people will tell you to take it easy for the first week or two after you give birth, but nobody tells you that the lochia flow is one good reason for this. Because your uterus hasn't healed yet, too much activity can cause excessive bleeding. I found this out the hard way.

Expect the lochia flow to get a little heavier whenever you increase your activity level, but gushing is a definite signal to slow down. (I remember wondering, when my own bleeding was so heavy, just how in the world, for the lochia reason alone, Olympian Mary Decker Slaney was able to start running again only *six days* after giving birth in 1986.)

Excessive bleeding (usually defined as saturating two or more pads in an hour) is only one lochia warning sign. Others that also necessitate a call to the doctor: passing large clots; seeing fresh red blood again after a period of rusty-colored discharge; discharge that itches, has a foul smell, or contains pus.

Your cervix will close. For the first-time mother in labor, it seems to take an eternity for the cervix to open to ten centimeters. After birth, it takes even longer (about ten days) for the cervix to close back down to normal. At least the closing process is painless!

You may suffer from hemorrhoids. My roommate in the hospital, who told me she hadn't suffered a single hemorrhoid during her pregnancy, got them in spades during the two hours it took her to push her baby out. As we lay there in our hospital beds that first night as new mothers, she was in agony. The hospital had given us little goody bags, and one of the products inside was diaper rash ointment. "I'll swap you this for a tube of Preparation H," my roommate would call to anyone who happened by, and she wasn't kidding.

For lots of reasons, pregnancy makes women more susceptible to hemorrhoids, the often painful, burning, itching, swollen veins that protrude from the anus. One is the immense pressure the growing fetus puts on the pelvic floor. Also, your blood supply increases, raising the pressure within the veins. Third, the constipation that may result from not drinking the additional liquids needed during pregnancy makes for hard, dry bowel movements that may need to be "strained" out—a practice that exacerbates hemorrhoids. And if you don't already have them when you go to deliver, you're very likely to develop them during the pushing stage of vaginal delivery. (If you had them during pregnancy, pushing will probably worsen them.) Seventy percent of women get hemorrhoids at some time during their pregnancy and/or delivery, according to the people at Preparation H. In Dwenda Gjerdingen's St. Paul, Minnesota, postpartum study, 29.3 percent of mothers who delivered vaginally were still bothered by hemorrhoids after one month, 14.8 percent at the three-month mark, and 11.2 percent at six. (Complaints about hemorrhoids were much lower among C-section mothers.)

You may have trouble urinating or having bowel movements. It takes about a month for the ureter and bladder— both of which are traumatized during pregnancy, labor, and delivery—to regain some semblance of their prepregnancy position and function. In the meantime, some women find urinating a little more of a chore than usual. If you have a cesarean section, in fact, you may need a catheter in your bladder for the first several postpartum days in order to empty it.

The bowel acts sluggish, too, because it lacks muscle tone in the first couple of postpartum months. Constipation is a very common problem among new mothers, especially in the first three weeks. It's harder to push out a bowel movement because the abdominal muscles are slack, and in C-section mothers those muscles have actually been cut. Lots of new moms dread moving their bowels anyway because they have hemorrhoids, or they fear they'll rupture episiotomy or C-section stitches (rare occurrences) or in the case of women who underwent C-sections it simply hurts to bear down. Delaying postpartum bowel movements, however, can cause constipation, and that just makes passing the wastes even more painful and difficult.

Your perineum will be sore. While she was pregnant, my friend Glenda read an article opposing routine episiotomy, the two- to four-centimeter cut that's made through the skin and muscle between the vagina and rectum to enlarge the vagina just before delivery. When Glenda's labor started and she went to the hospital, she was determined that she was not going to have one. " 'No episiotomy! No episiotomy!' I kept hissing that at my doctor instead of doing the breathing," she told me jokingly (I think). Well, Glenda had her way and didn't get an episiotomy. And she was astonished to find that her perineum was sore after birth anyway; she had difficulty sitting comfortably for days. She hadn't known that even if the perineum doesn't get cut or torn, it usually gets *bruised* during a vaginal delivery.

If you have an episiotomy, you will be even more uncomfortable. The most common episiotomy complaints during the first two weeks are pain, swelling, and itching. About 20 percent of women with episiotomies have problems with sexual intercourse for up to three months postpartum; about four in one hundred get an infection in the healing area.

Your breasts will become engorged. For the first couple of days after birth, your breasts will produce colostrum, the same nutrient-rich yellowish substance you may have occasionally noticed in the final weeks of pregnancy. If you're planning to breastfeed, the baby will subsist on colostrum in the first few days of life. At the colostrum stage, I remember thinking, This is a cinch! Why do people complain about it being hard to breastfeed?

On the third or fourth day after birth, you'll find your breasts swelling to a rock hardness as your real milk comes in. (Why does the milk always come in like clockwork regardless of whether your baby is born early, late, or on time? The current theory is that the placenta secretes hormones that suppress lactation and, once the placenta is out of you, it's no holds barred.) I will not kid you: engorgement is *very* uncomfortable. One of my friends told me she found the first few hours of engorgement as painful as labor, but I would not go *that* far (especially since that friend had an epidural). The worst of the engorgement discomfort is over within about twenty-four hours, and it will disappear completely in a few days as your milk supply adjusts to your baby's needs.

My own particular engorgement problem was that I swelled up so much I could not get my nipple into Madeline's tiny mouth. After several hot showers and lots of frantic pumping to no avail, I showed up at her pediatrician's office, a wild-eyed, Don King–haired, desperate woman toting a baby screaming with hunger. Wordlessly a nurse handed me a miraculous little device we came to fondly call "Mr. Nipple." It was simply a fake skinny nipple that covered my own until Madeline was big enough for the real thing.

A week or two into breastfeeding, you may find your nipples drying out, even cracking in places. Another not uncommon condition among breastfeeders (about 5 percent) is postpartum mastitis, an infection in one of the milk ducts. It's usually characterized by a hot and tender spot on the breast and a fever of up to 103 degrees. This kind of infection is treated with antibiotics, and there's no need to stop breastfeeding; your baby cannot "catch" the infection.

If you choose to bottle-feed instead of breastfeed, your milk will dry up in four to ten days. One mom I know who decided against nursing said that she wasn't as bothered by engorgement as she was by waking up every morning for the first week with dried milk on her nipples. This, she said, was very itchy and uncomfortable.

If you underwent a cesarean section, you will be recovering from major abdominal surgery. Look at it this way: When a woman has a hysterectomy, the surgeon cuts through the same muscles in the abdominal wall that are severed in a C-section—and that patient is typically excused from work for six to eight weeks in order to recover. The C-section mother does not have that luxury, however. She has a taxing, full-time job within *days* of her surgery.

My sister Sally, who's had three C-sections, remembers reading before her first that she'd have abdominal "discomfort" for only about three to five days. In actuality, she says, she was in a lot of pain for at least the first ten days and needed regular doses of prescription pain medication (Tylenol with codeine, as she recalls) throughout that period.

Two other C-section moms reported to me that the worst part of recovery for them wasn't pain in the incision area but the horrendous gas pains that hit within the first week after surgery. This gas is a product of trauma to the intestines, compounded by the fact that moms who have C-sections aren't able to move around very much for several days.

That's often another big surprise for women who have had C-sections: their lack of mobility. "The doctors give you a lot of prohibitions against driving and climbing stairs and that sort of thing," my sister said, "but you find you're also incapable of doing something as simple as sitting up in bed. In order to go to the bathroom, you have to prop yourself up on your arms and roll out of bed ... kind of the same way our Barbie dolls used to have to get up each morning."

Another common first-six-weeks-after-cesarean symptom I heard about was itchiness at the incision site. A few women told me they felt numb there, sometimes for months. One woman described the sensation she felt in her incision site, especially when she exercised or lay on her back, as "too tight—like a seam that's stretching to capacity." A more serious side effect of a C-section is infection. Some 20 to 40 percent of women who have the surgery suffer an infection, usually of the surgical wound, urinary tract, or uterus.

The good news for women who have cesarean rather than vaginal deliveries is that, according to that landmark St. Paul study I keep mentioning, they have far fewer problems in the first postpartum year with certain physical ailments (such as acne, hemorrhoids, vaginal discomfort, discomfort with intercourse, and difficulty reaching orgasm) than women do who have vaginal deliveries.

The pounds will drop off. The average woman who gains twenty-five to thirty-five pounds during pregnancy can expect to drop about fifteen of those immediately after delivery. That's the weight of the baby, the placenta, and amniotic fluid. In the first couple of weeks after delivery, you'll drop another five to ten pounds.

But you will still probably look pregnant. One of my friends told me that when her in-laws arrived at the hospital to pay her and her baby their first postpartum visit, she was standing at the window. Her father-in-law took one look at her and cracked, "So when is the baby due?" My friend burst into tears.

Don't expect an instant hard body upon delivery and absolutely do not make the mistake of bequeathing all of your maternity clothes to a pregnant friend as you leave for the hospital. Because of your still-enlarged uterus and your slackened abdominal muscles, at the very least your postpartum stomach will look loose and flabby for a while—a deflated basketball is an apt description—and a couple of mothers I interviewed admitted to looking six or seven months pregnant for several weeks after birth. My sister Sally, who has had several babies, says her abdomen always looked pretty good right after delivery but then poofed back out a few days later when the postcesarean gas hit.

You may sweat profusely. A major part of those five to ten pounds that come off so easily in the first week is water weight. About twelve hours after birth, via increased perspiration and urination, the body begins to flush out all the extra fluids it's been carrying. Usually the increased perspiration ends six to eight weeks after birth. For my friend Roberta, however, it lasted up to a year after each of her three children was born. She feels this was at least partially due to the fact that she breastfed each of those babies for several months and "bigger breasts make you sweat more."

Increased thirst is common because your body wants to replace some of the fluid you're losing. You may also have night sweats and hot flashes (usually thought of as symptoms of menopause) because estrogen levels plummet after birth. Hot flashes are particularly common when a breastfeeding mother's milk first "lets down" at the beginning of a nursing session. The St. Paul postpartum study found that about 10 percent of the new mothers were still having hot flashes at one month postpartum.

You may begin menstruating. If you're not breastfeeding, you'll probably begin menstruating again after two or three months. In breastfeeding women, ovulation is hormonally suppressed, but probably *not* for the entire time you breast-feed. In a recent study at the Johns Hopkins Medical Institutions, researchers found that several factors—mostly frequency, duration, and intensity of nursing—determine when you'll become fertile again. As you begin tapering your baby off the breast and onto other foods, your chances of ovulating steadily rise. The guesstimate usually given to nursing mothers about when their first period will occur is six to eight months after childbirth. Keep in mind there's tremendous variation possible here; one nursing mom told me she got her period back only six weeks after she delivered. (That's extremely rare, however. The Johns Hopkins study found that only 3 percent of breastfeeding mothers ovulated during the second month postpartum.)

Another thing to keep in mind is that you don't have to have a menstrual period before your first ovulation occurs. In other words, use birth control unless you like the idea of children spaced only twelve or fifteen months apart. I have seen statistics that the chances of conceiving again within a year of childbirth are 90 percent for a nonbreastfeeding woman who doesn't use birth control and 40 percent for her breastfeeding counterpart.

Expect your first period after childbirth to be weird in some way: lighter or heavier than usual; longer or shorter than what you were used to. My own first postpartum period stood out because it was the only one I've ever had that wasn't accompanied by cramps. You should start getting back into a regular pattern with the second period.

Your lower back will probably ache. During pregnancy
your center of gravity changes—it moves forward as your
abdomen and breasts steadily enlarge. This causes you to
arch or sway your back. If you don't suffer backaches
during pregnancy, there's a better than even chance that
you will postpartum; *Parents* magazine says 60 percent of
new mothers do. Not only will your back be struggling to
adjust to the new dynamics of your nonpregnant body,
your slackened abdominal muscles won't be providing
much if any back support, and you'll aggravate these conditions by doing a lot of lifting (of the baby) and leaning or
bending (over the crib, the changing table, the car seat).

You may be battling acne. In the last two trimesters of
pregnancy, many acne-prone women see an improvement
in their complexions because their hormone levels are so in
sync. After the baby is born, however, these same women
suffer breakouts for several weeks or even months because
of fluctuating hormonal levels combined with the stress of
caring for a new baby (stress is a major cause of acne in
adults).

In the St. Paul postpartum study, 16.8 percent of the new
moms who delivered vaginally had acne at one month
postpartum, and 13.4 had it at three months. In cesarean
moms, the numbers were 11.5 and 6.4 percent, respec-
tively. Dwenda Gjerdingen, the study leader, says she can't
explain why the cesarean moms had less acne.

Fatigue will set in. Whenever one of my sisters or friends
would have a baby, I used to wait a full twenty-four hours
after birth to call the hospital, figuring that the new
mother would be absolutely comatose for hours after birth,
thanks to the rigors of labor and delivery. Then I had my
own child. Now I call mothers on the very first night,

figuring there's a terrific chance they have insomnia, just like I did.

The nurses at my hospital told me that insomnia the first night after birth is common, even if the new mother got little or no sleep the *previous* night because of labor. You can be just too revved up with excitement and joy. After-birth insomnia is particularly common in first-time mothers, but experienced two- and three-timers undergo it, too. My friend Roberta, who worked in a bank's corporate offices, completed her department's annual budget during the night following her second child's birth.

A lot of mothers told me that they also felt positively terrific and superenergized on the second or even the third day after birth. I was one of these myself. Boy, did I think I was hot stuff. I had my baby on Thursday night; left the hospital on Friday afternoon; and on Saturday attended two baby showers (for me), did a week's worth of grocery shopping, and took Madeline to the pediatrician to have her jaundice checked.

On Sunday, I absolutely crashed and burned—and bled like crazy. I was so tired and weak that I had to psyche myself up for several minutes before moving from my chair to my bed. This crash, too, I have learned, is the common experience of women who begin parenthood high on adrenaline.

Expect fatigue to set in, whether it's three minutes or three days after childbirth. "I remember one time during the first week when I tottered to the bathroom like an old lady," a friend told me. "I had to grab onto things along the way. Then I got up from the toilet and saw stars. And here I'd been a woman who'd exercised and stayed in shape throughout my pregnancy and had a relatively short, uncomplicated labor and delivery, no epidural, not even an episiotomy. It was ridiculous."

But it *isn't* ridiculous. Not when you combine the rigors of labor and delivery with the physically taxing breakneck pace at which your body is changing, and then throw in the sleep deprivation that comes with the necessity of feeding a newborn every 2½ or 3 hours. Postpartum side effects such as constipation, sweating, and thirst also contribute to fatigue.

Well, here I am, supposedly the great cheerleader of the wonders of motherhood, and I just spent pages and pages on stuff that might best be described with a word you'll soon hear regularly: *yucky*. Believe me, it gets better in the next chapter. In the meantime, however, there are a couple of things to keep in mind as you hobble around wearing an ice pack, Preparation H, a saddle-sized sanitary napkin below the belt, and a soggy nursing bra and/or sweaty, radically shifting nursing pads above it. First, unlike with most physical sufferings, such as the flu or a broken arm, you get a fabulous reward in return, and that's the baby, of course. When a friend read that last sentence, she had this comment: "Now wait a minute. Let's just be frank. In the first few weeks, you may not think that baby is so fabulous. He or she may be little more to you than a red-faced little blob who is either constantly latched onto your body or squalling to high heaven. Before you know it, however, he'll be gazing up at you with adoring eyes, lighting up like a Christmas tree whenever you enter the room, maybe even laughing at your jokes. That stuff makes *this* stuff worth it."

The other thing to keep in mind is that *these* transitions, at least, are only *temporary*. It may help to repeat to yourself what Ann Landers calls the four most comforting words in the universe: "This, too, shall pass." It really does.

Okay—But How Do You Define "Temporary"?

Doctors have traditionally labeled the first six weeks after birth the "postpartum recovery period" because that's how long it takes for the reproductive organs to return to their nonpregnant state. But evidence is mounting that it takes many women a good deal longer than that before they feel like their old selves or, as I like to put it, before they feel new and improved. In the St. Paul study—I've sprinkled statistics from it throughout this chapter—a significant percentage of women were still experiencing childbirth-related problems such as hemorrhoids, vaginal discomfort, and discomfort with intercourse at six and even twelve months postpartum.

In another study—this one conducted in the late 1980s by registered nurses Lorraine Tulman, Ph.D., and Jacqueline Fawcett, Ph.D., of the University of Pennsylvania (Philadelphia) School of Nursing—only 51 percent of seventy women surveyed said they had regained their usual energy by six weeks postpartum. Even at six *months* postpartum, 25 percent of the new mothers said they did not feel physically recovered, and they reported problems with lack of sleep, fatigue, and difficulty losing weight, as well as emotional concerns such as mood swings and dealing with increased responsibilities. In that study, the women most frequently pointed to prolonged labor and/or cesarean delivery as the biggest hindrances to recovery.

And here's one more study to shore up your confidence in yourself if you're not one of those women who bounce right back to normal within a few weeks of birth. When the Melpomene Institute for Women's Health Research in Minneapolis asked a group of new mothers whether they

felt fully recovered or back to "being themselves" two
months after giving birth, only 50 percent of the women
the Institute categorized as nonathletic answered yes. More
significantly, among new mothers who were athletes, only
53 percent of the runners and 60 percent of the swimmers
Melpomene studied answered that question in the affirma-
tive. And these were women whose preconception and
pregnancy fitness levels would tend, one would assume, to
make their postpartum physical recovery easier in many
respects.

The point here is that you should not get down on
yourself or even be very surprised if your recovery actually
takes longer than the six weeks typically stipulated by
doctors and employers. Try some of the suggestions in the
first several pages of Chapter 3 for coping in the first
several weeks, but *see your doctor* about physical problems
that persist beyond the first two months. Be assertive about
getting these problems fixed once and for all. I personally
hounded my HMO till I got my episiotomy surgically
repaired. A friend with postpartum hemorrhoids, fed up
with her doctor's "prescriptions" of sitz baths and Preparation H, had them surgically removed. Said she: "I hate that
Preparation H commercial where the guy comes home
from the doctor and says something like 'Great news, hon.
The doctor says I don't need surgery on my hemorrhoids.'
What that commercial doesn't tell you is that without the
surgery that guy is probably going to have to go around for
the rest of his life greased with Preparation H. Well, I for
one decided I was not going to support that company for
the rest of my life!"

And on that note, let us go on to, well, not necessarily
bigger but certainly better things.

CHAPTER TWO

YOUR BODY, ONLY DIFFERENT

What You Can Expect from the "New You"

The first six weeks aside, pregnancy and childbirth leave lasting and often permanent changes to the body. Let us count the ways . . .

The Organs in the Birth Area

The uterus. Even after involution (postpartum shrinking), the uterus of a mother will forever after remain a little larger than it was prior to pregnancy. The difference in size isn't perceptible to us, but it's enough to enable a doctor who performs pelvic exams to tell who's given birth and who hasn't.

The *position* of the uterus is also different in a woman who has given birth. As the uterus grows during pregnancy, it stretches the pelvic tissues and ligaments that support it (and the bladder and rectum), and this support system gets a further workout if a woman delivers vaginally. Though the body repairs tissues and ligaments to some extent after birth, some pelvic relaxation (as it's known in the industry) is permanent. "The uterus will forever ride lower than it did before pregnancy," according to Stephen DiMarzo, M.D., a La Jolla, California, obstetrician and gynecologist (OB/GYN). "How much lower depends on the stretching that occurred, and that is determined in large part by the size of the baby, the length and difficulty of the labor and delivery, and—of course—whether the birth was vaginal or by C-section," he said. "Genetics play a role in this, too. The strength and resiliency of the ligaments are inherited."

The extreme version of this drop in the position of the uterus is called a prolapse. In this rare condition, the uterus sinks into the vagina and causes problems. "Prolapse patients are almost always women who have had several vaginal births, not just one or two," said DiMarzo.

The bladder and rectum. The stretching of the pelvic support mechanisms can also affect the position and function of the bladder and rectum. One common result is reduced bladder capacity, such as that being experienced by my friend Gail, who has had to get up two times every night since she was seven months pregnant—three years ago. But Nancy Cetel, M.D., an Encinitas, California, physician specializing in women's health once suggested to me that some cases like Gail's may in fact be based on new habits rather than on physical necessity. In the last few weeks of pregnancy, most of us become accustomed to having to get up a few times a night because our bladders are so squeezed they're incapable of holding more than a few teaspoonfuls of urine. The get-up-and-go habit may become even more deeply ingrained after birth, according to Cetel. "You get so used to getting up for feedings that getting up becomes a part of your routine," she said.

DiMarzo said that an even more common complaint

than reduced bladder capacity is not having the same prebaby ability to hold urine—also known as stress incontinence (or, as one of my friends puts it, the "leak-when-you-laugh syndrome"). The more the bladder and its supporting structures are traumatized during pregnancy and delivery—which is in large part determined by the size of the baby—the greater the likelihood you'll later suffer bouts of stress incontinence. All indications are that eating too much during pregnancy makes the baby big, and pushing that big baby out is the number one culprit with this kind of trouble. Cetel added that sometimes—though rarely after only one or two vaginal births—the wall between the vagina and the rectum remains "relaxed," so that a woman will have more difficulty producing bowel movements than she did prior to having a baby.

The labia. Social anthropologist and childbirth educator Sheila Kitzinger said in *The Complete Book of Pregnancy and Childbirth* that after you've had a baby your labia, "like the outside petals of a flower, are softer and fleshier" than they were prebaby. We'll just have to take her word for it, since—as liberated as we're supposed to be—I was unable to find a mom who would admit to having anything more than a passing acquaintance with the looks of her prebaby labia. Maybe our daughters will be different. The editor of an East Coast parenting magazine told me her four-year-old daughter takes a hand mirror and stares, transfixed, at her genitalia for a half-hour or more. "I myself had never done that," said the editor, "until I went into labor."

The cervix. A doctor performing a pelvic exam can tell whether or not a patient has ever borne children just by looking at her cervix (the opening of the uterus). The cervix of a woman who has not had a child is very tiny; generally, that of a mother is larger and irregularly shaped (one reason to have a diaphragm refitted after birth). The change in shape exposes more glands along the cervical canal in some women, giving them a heavier day-to-day vaginal discharge than they had prepregnancy. Two women told me they are very thankful for this because it's now much easier for them to tell when they are ovulating. When cervical mucus turns "fertile"—that is, when it becomes stretchy and egg-white–like just before and during ovulation to facilitate the sperm's journey to the egg—it's much more copious and evident in these two women than it was prechildren.

Doctors used to think that this new larger cervix was responsible for the fact that most women have less intense menstrual cramps after pregnancy than they did before. The theory was that because the opening of the cervix is bigger, the uterus doesn't have to work so hard—cramp, in other words—to expel the blood. *Wrong!* (See "Menstrual Periods" in this chapter.)

The vagina. If you deliver vaginally, the vagina, which is stretched to capacity during delivery, gradually regains most of its prepregnancy muscle tone in the first two months after birth. "A lot of women think that after they have an eight-pound baby they'll literally have an eight-pound tunnel between their legs," Fritzi Kallop, R.N., a nationally known childbirth educator and author of *Fritzi Kallop's Birth Book*, once told me. "But the vagina does heal back down." In other words, your husband will still be able to feel you and you will still be able to feel your husband.

The vagina, however, will usually remain a little larger than it was before pregnancy, another reason why it's important to be refitted for a diaphragm after giving birth. "Most women will feel as if they are a little looser, but not noticeably enough to decrease sexual pleasure either for themselves or for their partners," said OB/GYN DiMarzo.

The Breasts

According to Susan Love, M.D., the UCLA breast surgeon who wrote *Dr. Susan Love's Breast Book*, in a purely technical sense your breasts aren't fully mature until you've given birth and produced milk. "The breasts of women who do not give birth remain in the earlier stage of development until menopause," Love wrote.

So, hurrah! We've got mature breasts! But there's a depressing-sounding term for what happens to most of our mature breasts after a baby: *postpartum atrophy*. It's responsible for the fact that almost every mother I interviewed for this book reported that her breasts ended up smaller—as much as a cup size—than they were prepregnancy, once she was finished with pregnancy, childbirth, and breastfeeding. Here's how James Pietraszek, M.D., a La Jolla, California, plastic surgeon, explained it to me. During pregnancy the breasts enlarge, but after the baby is born (or after we quit nursing) the breasts, which have been waiting around since puberty to provide milk, lose fatty tissue; it simply atrophies away.

We're also likely to sag more after pregnancy and childbirth. For one thing, the skin envelope that holds the now-diminished breast tissue is stretched out from the enlargement of the breasts during pregnancy. But the major blame for the sag factor lies with the Cooper's ligaments (also known as the suspensory ligaments), the strands of fibrous tissue that encase and support the entire breast and that stretch to accommodate breast growth during pregnancy.

They are not elastic and never regain their original shape, according to San Diego surgeon Sheryl Cramer, M.D. Obviously, the potential for sagging is even greater if you breastfeed, since the breasts remain enlarged longer. And, according to Cramer (70 to 80 percent of whose surgeries involve the breast), you get progressively saggier and smaller with each baby. "I have a friend who once wore a C cup, but now, after three kids, she no longer wears a bra at all," Cramer said. "She says, 'Why bother, with a AA?' "

Some experts recommend keeping a pillow under your baby while she is nursing in order to support her head and reduce the chances of her pulling down on the breasts. It's also a good idea to wear a supportive bra as much as possible—even while you sleep and especially while exercising—during pregnancy and in the postpartum weeks or months of nursing. "This will save some of your elasticity, but some will go no matter what you do," according to Cramer. (See Chapter 6 for tips on buying maternity and nursing bras.)

It's not *all* bad news. Pregnancy and breastfeeding help decrease your odds of getting breast cancer (see "Female Cancers" in this chapter). And Cramer says that once you have a baby your mammograms are easier to read. That's because pregnancy, as explained, uses up some of the glandular breast tissue. This tissue shows up white and dense on mammograms and makes cancers harder to detect.

And here's a real stunner: Once you've had a baby, you can always breastfeed in the future even if you never give birth again, according to Susan Love. If you adopt a baby, for example, and the baby sucks your breast long enough, the whole milk-producing process will kick into gear again. Evidently, prolactin (the hormone produced by the pituitary gland that triggers the production of milk) is always present in the pituitary, but substances secreted by the hypothalamus in the brain keep it from being secreted until after you've been through a pregnancy (although there have been rare cases of women who have not given birth gaining the ability to lactate).

Menstrual Periods

The majority of mothers I interviewed noticed some change in their menstrual periods—in comparison to pre-baby days—after pregnancy, delivery, and breastfeeding. Mostly I heard a triumphant "My cramps aren't as bad as they were before the baby" or even "I don't get cramps anymore."

Doctors used to believe this big benefit of childbearing could be attributed to the fact that a woman's cervix is bigger after she gives birth. Because of this, so the theory went, the uterus doesn't have to contract (cramp) so hard in order to expel the menstrual blood. Many doctors—and that includes many gynecologists—*still* believe this.

Then how do they account for moms like me, whose cramps are every bit as bad as ever? Or, if I'm some sort of exception because I only had one baby, how does the theory explain the bone-crushing cramps of my two sisters, each of whom has given birth to three large babies? Or of my mother, who had four? Just how large does that puppy have to get before you can expect some relief?

Neysa Whiteman, M.D., is one gynecologist who agrees with me that the new, improved, family-size cervix is taking credit where credit is not due. "If the stretched-cervix theory were true, then every childless woman who has her cervix dilated—say, for an abortion or a D and C [dilation and curettage]—would also see a reduction in cramps during her menstrual periods, and that's just not the case," Whiteman said. "Then, too, I've seen women whose cervixes look like pinholes, yet who don't have cramps at all."

I found an article written by Stanley J. Birnbaum, M.D., the chief of gynecology at New York Hospital, that offers a much more plausible explanation of why some women get less painful menstrual cramps once they've had a baby. Birnbaum said that because ovulation is suspended so long during pregnancy (and breastfeeding), when it begins again it is at a new hormonal level. Birnbaum believes that periods are usually less painful after childbirth because these hormonal changes may affect "the level or type of prostaglandins secreted by the endometrium [uterine lining]." (Prostaglandins are a group of hormones that cause the uterus to contract, and they can also cause, besides cramping, the nausea, fluid retention, diarrhea, and other menstrual problems some women have.) According to Birnbaum, the theory is that women who have bad menstrual cramps either secrete more prostaglandins or are just more sensitive to them than women who don't experience cramps. And this doesn't necessarily change after pregnancy.

Birnbaum said that the new hormonal levels after pregnancy may also result in an entirely new menstrual pattern, such as more or fewer days of bleeding and longer or shorter times between periods.

The Skin

Abdominal skin. Skin is more elastic than muscle. That's why the skin across the abdomen does a much better and quicker job than the abdominal muscles of snapping back to a prepregnancy state on its own. Most of us, however, will forevermore have looser abdominal skin than we did prepregnancy. The degree of looseness depends both on how much the skin had to stretch to accommodate the fetus and on the elasticity of your particular skin, which is determined by genetics and age (skin loses elasticity as it ages).

Stretch marks. "Stretch marks, unfortunately, are permanent," said Leslie Mark, M.D., a San Diego dermatologist. "While the red color will gradually fade to a normal skin tone, the indentations are there to stay." Mark said that whether or not you get stretch marks is determined partly by how much the skin has to stretch during pregnancy but also by your genes. "Some women," she said, "gain seventy-five pounds without a mark." Actress Susan Sarandon, by the way, told the *Los Angeles Times* that she doesn't have stretch marks "probably because I was so old when I had my kids there was nothing left to stretch." And she may have something there. A recent study on stretch marks at St. Paul–Ramsey Medical Center in St. Paul, Minnesota, found that women with abdominal stretch marks were significantly *younger* than their stretch mark–free counterparts. This study also found that women with abdominal stretch marks had—no surprise—a greater total pregnancy weight gain than did women without and, intriguingly, were more likely to receive state medical assistance. Diane J. Madlon-Kay, M.D., one of the study's leaders, said this latter factor was "presumably because such women have a low-protein diet and, therefore, poorer connective tissue formation."

Leslie Mark said that, contrary to popular belief, rubbing on Vitamin E oil or a similar lubricating product during pregnancy may make your skin feel better but it won't prevent stretch marks. "The fibers that are stretching are in the deeper layers of the skin, where creams can't penetrate," she said.

Yes, but maybe Retin-A *can*, according to Chula Vista, California, dermatologist Peter Rullan, M.D. Like most physicians, he believes pregnant women should not use Retin-A. But he said there has been a French study supported by some U.S. studies showing that if you apply Retin-A to stretch marks early on—right after the baby is born, when the marks are still pink and fresh—there's a 50 percent or greater chance that you'll see significant improvement.

Pigment changes. High hormonal levels during pregnancy are responsible for two pigment-related skin changes: the linea nigra, a thin, dark line that runs up the center of the abdomen, and the mask of pregnancy, a series of brownish stains across the forehead, cheeks, and nose (women who get a lot of sun exposure during pregnancy are particularly prone to this). Most cases of both of these will clear up in the six months after delivery, according to Mark. Rullan said that pigmentation can occasionally act like a permanent tattoo; he's seen women who need professional help to rid themselves of these pregnancy pigmentation problems long after they've given birth. He said they can be very successfully treated by dermatologists with bleaching agents, chemical peels, or both.

Moles and other growths. During pregnancy, the pregnancy hormones also make our epidermal growth factor—the protein that stimulates things to grow on the skin—more active, said Rullan. The most potentially serious consequence is that, according to a recent study, precancerous changes in moles develop almost four times as fast when we're pregnant as when we're not. (Report any mole changes to your OB/GYN immediately.) My friend Roberta developed two entirely *new* moles, one on each breast, during her second pregnancy. The growth factor also causes many women to develop fibroepithelial polyps, commonly known as skin tags, or the ones they had before pregnancy grow even bigger, said Rullan. Common areas for these benign and usually painless annoyances: on the neck, under the arms, around the eyes. Rullan said these polyps do not disappear after pregnancy, and many women seek their removal (via excision or a very light laser burn) simply because they consider the tags unsightly.

Rullan added that the pregnancy hormones, coupled with increased blood flow to the skin during pregnancy, can be blamed for the little red "blood moles" that develop on the trunk. Blood moles are officially known as cherry angiomas and, like skin tags, they are benign and removable with professional help.

Perioral dermatitis. Thanks again to hormones, or so the theory goes, many women get their first case of perioral dermatitis during pregnancy. This ugly red rash around the mouth and chin is frequently mistaken for acne. But it is not acne; acne cures, in fact, seem to make it worse. In nonpregnant women, the rash can be successfully cleared up with oral tetracycline. Pregnant women, who can't take tetracycline because it's believed to affect the bones and teeth of the developing fetus, are often given oral or topical erythromycin for the problem. These medications, however, don't appear to cure the problem permanently. The skin is still prone to flare-ups for six months to two years after the initial outbreak.

Teeth and Gums

High levels of progesterone during pregnancy can alter the blood vessels of your mouth, increasing your chances of getting gingivitis or making the gingivitis you had prepregnancy even worse, according to Barbara J. Steinberg, D.D.S., a professor of dental medicine at the Medical College of Pennsylvania in Philadelphia. Thirty to 60 percent of pregnant women develop gingivitis, which is an early stage of periodontal (gum) disease caused by plaque—a sticky mix of mucus, bacteria, and food that forms at the base of a tooth. The telltale signs of gingivitis are red, puffy gums that bleed easily.

The peak period for pregnancy gingivitis, according to Steinberg, is between the second and eighth months. The inflammation declines throughout the postpartum months as hormone levels return to normal.

Steinberg said that the elevated hormonal levels of pregnancy do not themselves cause gingivitis. "There's usually a cofactor involved," she said, "and the most salient contributing factor is poor oral hygiene." She did add, however, that in some women the hormonal factors play the greatest role, and she named herself as an example. She said she had gingivitis while pregnant even though she was—as one might expect—fastidious about her oral hygiene.

Steinberg said such fastidiousness, which includes brushing and flossing religiously and getting regular professional cleanings throughout your pregnancy, is the best insurance that gingivitis won't become a permanent souvenir of pregnancy. This regimen keeps the gingivitis of most women under control, but some women, said Steinberg, may still require corrective surgery after the postpartum period. The surgery involves cleaning out all the inflammatory tissue.

Steinberg said another dental problem some women get while pregnant is called a pregnancy tumor, or epulis. This benign lesion, which occurs on the gum where it comes to a point between two teeth, is another product of high hormone levels and plaque. The tumor looks like a big gum boil, can bleed easily, and may have to be excised during pregnancy. Otherwise, the tumor generally just disappears after childbirth. "Sometimes, though, the gum still has to be recontoured by a dentist; that is, gum surgery may be required in order to restore the normal configuration of the gum," Steinberg said.

I told Steinberg that a fellow writer had said her dentist insists that women who have given birth need much more Novocain to numb their gums during dental work than women who haven't. In fact, this dentist said many mothers simply can't be numbed no matter how much Novocain they're given. Steinberg had never heard of that.

She said a much more common old husbands' tale is that "for every child a tooth is lost." "It used to be believed that if a fetus needed calcium it was taken from the mother's teeth, but that's not true," according to Steinberg. "If calcium has to be liberated from the mother's body, it would have to come from her bones, but even that's a rarity, especially in America. Most women here eat decently and are not nutritionally deprived. The fetus can thrive on the calcium that the mother ingests from food."

The only real way to lose teeth during pregnancy is to let gingivitis get out of hand, said Steinberg, and that just doesn't have to happen.

Eyes

Optometrists don't want to fit pregnant women for new contact lenses. This is because hormonal changes can temporarily alter the shape of the cornea, so the lenses might not fit after the baby is born. Joseph Shovlin, an optometrist in Scranton, Pennsylvania, and the past chairman of the Contact Lens Section of the American Optometric Association, suggests that women wait at least six months after birth to get first-time contacts.

What if you're already a contact lens wearer when you get pregnant? Shovlin, who is also on the Food and Drug Administration's Ophthalmic Devices Panel and the National Institutes of Health's National Advisory Council, said that the majority of patients who wear *soft* lenses during pregnancy shouldn't have any problem with the eye changes of pregnancy, which, besides the alteration of the cornea (generally, its shape steepens), usually also include a decrease in the production of tear film. Some rigid contact lens wearers, on the other hand, may develop an intolerance, according to Shovlin. "That's why we always recommend that pregnant women have a pair of glasses with an updated prescription, just in case," he said.

He said eyes should be back to their prepregnancy state six to nine months after birth (longer if you nurse, because breastfeeding keeps hormone levels elevated). Is there a chance your eyes will be *permanently* altered by your pregnancy? Shovlin said he has not seen or heard of a case like that in his twelve years of practice.

Feet

I have a friend whose mother insists she grew a half shoe size every time she had a baby. She started, prebabies, with size 7 feet; after bearing four children, she now wears size 9s. This was my experience exactly. Before Madeline, I wore a size 8½; after the sixth month of my pregnancy, I went up a size to 9 and have stayed that size ever since. I was stunned to learn this experience is more the rule than the exception.

"As people get older in general, their foot size tends to

enlarge, both in width and length," said Glenn Gastwirth, D.P.M., deputy executive director of the American Podiatric Medical Association. "This is because of all the weight that's put on the feet while we walk and stand over the years. They just stretch out."

During pregnancy, said Gastwirth, this process speeds up, not just because of the extra weight that's being put on the feet but also because the body is circulating the pregnancy hormone known as relaxin. Relaxin's specific job is to relax the connective and supportive tissue around the fetus, so that fetal growth can be accommodated and birth will be made easier. But relaxin affects supportive tissue throughout the entire body, including the ligaments and tendons that hold and maintain structure in the feet.

Hair

If your hair feels thicker and more luxuriant during pregnancy, you're not dreaming. It *is*. In the second half of pregnancy, hormonal influences apparently alter the normal pattern of hair growth. Usually, hair has a resting phase, when existing hairs die and are shed, and a growing phase, when new hairs replace the shed ones. During pregnancy, high estrogen levels extend the growing cycle and prevent the resting cycle.

About two or three months after the baby is born, the scalp makes up for lost time by shedding many more hairs than during a normal resting cycle. (The physical stress of labor and delivery and the anesthesia used during a C-section are also believed to exacerbate postpartum hair loss.) In most new mothers, the shedding is minimal—five hundred to six hundred hairs a day is average. This sounds terrible unless you know that we normally lose a couple hundred hairs a day anyway. Janet Rogers, M.D., a clinical professor of dermatology at the Oregon Health Sciences University in Portland, told *Parents* magazine that a small number of women lose a significant amount of hair—up to 40 percent of their hair, in fact. Rogers said that, in any case, while postpartum hair loss comes from the entire scalp, the majority is lost around the hairline and can extend two or three inches into the crown area.

Fortunately, the loss is temporary. One finding of the landmark 1989 study of 436 first-time mothers in St. Paul, Minnesota, was that hair loss peaked at six months postpartum (that's when the growing phase typically begins again), then declined over the next six months.

Most women will eventually end up with the same amount of hair they had prior to getting pregnant. However, Philip Kingsley, a London and New York City expert on hair and its diseases, told *Redbook* magazine that "I've noticed that women who have been through multiple pregnancies seem to wind up with thinner hair [for good]."

You have probably heard women say that their wavy hair lost its curl—or their straight hair turned curly—after they gave birth. While I could find no studies on this phenomenon, it seems logical that it must have something to do with the shock to the body caused by pregnancy and childbirth. One fact that leads me to believe this is that a friend who underwent chemotherapy, a process that is similarly stressful to the body, also reported a permanent change in her hair (in her case, she went from curly to straight).

Veins

As discussed in Chapter 1, pregnancy and childbirth are prime times for hemorrhoids. "Typically, hemorrhoids shrink within a few weeks after birth," Encinitas, California, physician Nancy Cetel told me, "but they often don't disappear completely." She did say that if you have hemorrhoids removed, you *won't* be more susceptible to hemorrhoids in the future than someone who has never had them. (See Chapter 3 for more on coping with/curing these annoying "rosettes," as Cetel wryly refers to them.)

Another souvenir of pregnancy may be varicose veins in the legs. About one in four pregnant women gets varicose veins, which develop when valves that run the length of the major saphenous vein give out, trapping blood in the lower extremities. The blood presses on the walls of the valves and causes them to swell. All of the pregnancy-related factors that make pregnant women more susceptible to hemorrhoids—pressure, expanding blood supply, constipation—also make them more susceptible to varicose veins. (A hemorrhoid is, essentially, a varicose vein in the anus.)

Sometimes the only problem with varicose veins is cosmetic: they look ugly. But in more severe cases, they can make your legs feel tired and achy. As with hemorrhoids, varicose veins tend to improve after childbirth, but they usually persist, and subsequent pregnancies exacerbate them. For example, by her third pregnancy, one of my sisters was having to wiggle into heavy elastic stockings every morning when she got out of bed. (See Chapter 3 for more info on coping/curing.)

In some women, but usually only those who have had several children, the pelvic veins become enlarged and varicose-like during pregnancy and stay that way, resulting in swelling of the pelvic tissues. The condition, called pelvic congestion syndrome, can hurt, and the pain often worsens during sex, walking, or bending forward.

Spider veins—technically known as spider angiomas— are fine, dilated blood vessels that often show up during pregnancy on the face, neck, chest, hands, and arms.

They're the result of elevated estrogen levels and usually go away after childbirth. If yours don't, see Chapter 3.

Fat and Weight

Former supermodel Patti Hansen (now married to Rolling Stone Keith Richards) told a *Mirabella* magazine writer that her body has gotten better after having two kids. "It just moved around in the right places," she said. "The lines changed." I remember reading somewhere that actress Cheryl Ladd was also thrilled with her postbaby body. She had considered her prepregnancy figure too boyish and loved it that having children had given her some hips. On the other hand, former "Dallas" actress Victoria Principal once told *Redbook* that "it would not be in my best physical interest to have a baby, so I've made the decision not to have any." And according to the *Los Angeles Times Magazine*, doctors at the Institute for Reproductive Research at the Hospital of the Good Samaritan in Los Angeles have turned down the requests of actresses, "who wanted to stay eligible for juicy roles," for embryo transfers—that is, to have their own embryos transferred into the wombs of other women willing to carry the resulting fetus to term for a fee.

Apparently, what all these women are worried about or thankful for is pregnancy's propensity for adding *fat*. During pregnancy, Mother Nature and hormonal changes direct that if a woman doesn't already have extra fatty tissue, such stores must be accumulated. Why? "Probably because in the dim dark past of prehistoric times, women who weren't able to eat enough and didn't have stored energy weren't successful reproducers. Their babies were too light in weight to survive," said Rose Frisch, the Harvard reproductive biologist who has been called "the chief student of female fat" in the United States. Voila! Mothers got fat reserves, and evolution hasn't yet caught up with the fact that food is now readily available and right around the corner at the supermarket.

Of course, you can limit the amount of fat you put on during pregnancy by being careful about the quantity and quality of food you eat (see Chapters 3 and 6 for more on this). But all pregnant women should resign themselves to the fact that they'll be gaining at least some new fat— about four kilograms (8.82 pounds) is average, according to Frisch—and most of that will go on the hips, thighs, and buttocks. Your postpartum metabolism will burn off some or maybe even most of that in the weeks or months after childbirth.

Keep in mind that the average woman gains twenty-five to thirty-five pounds during her pregnancy. The usual rule of thumb is that fifteen pounds of that will come off the day you deliver and you'll drop another five to ten pounds in the first couple of weeks without even trying. Whatever's left is body fat that needs to be worked off.

Who sheds pregnancy weight the fastest? This is an area fraught with conflicting studies. Kathryn Dewey, a professor of nutrition at the University of California at Davis, says that breastfeeding women do. Dewey studied eighty-seven women—about half of them breastfeeders—for a year after they gave birth. She found that the nursers lost twice as much postpregnancy weight (ten pounds) as the bottle-feeding moms (five pounds).

But in another recent study, researchers did *not* find breastfeeding beneficial for weight loss. Charles W. Schauberger, M.D., an OB/GYN at the Gundersen Clinic in La Crosse, Wisconsin, and his associates followed almost eight hundred women for six months postpartum. Two-thirds of these women were breastfeeding at the beginning

of the study; less than a fifth were still breastfeeding at
six months.

The researchers found that the sooner women returned
to work outside the home, the more weight they lost. "This
is probably due to greater physical activity and less access
to food on the job," Schauberger told *Redbook*. He went on
to speculate that his team found no link between breastfeeding and weight loss because "women who are breastfeeding need to eat well, and it may even be that the
hormones that induce lactation also stimulate appetite."

Other factors the La Crosse team found unlikely to
affect weight loss: the mother's age, use of oral contracep-
tives, alcohol consumption, marital status, and amount of
exercise. The study found that 22 percent of the mothers
lost all their pregnancy weight by six weeks postpartum,
37 percent had done so by six months, and the remaining
41 percent were still carrying extra weight at six months.
First-time mothers lost the most weight. This jibes with
another statistic that I came across: mothers gain, and keep,
an average of five pounds for each child.

There's long been a popular belief among new mothers
that fat gained during pregnancy is somehow different
from other body fat and is therefore more difficult to shed.
Experts have for just as long pooh-poohed this belief.
When I mentioned it to one expert in 1990 while putting
together an article on this same subject, she said, "The
chemical structure of pregnancy fat is exactly the same as
all other fat." Another expert—agreeing with the first—
told me he believed the real reason new moms have difficulty ridding themselves of pregnancy fat is that they don't
have enough time or energy to work out and to plan, shop
for, and cook healthy, low-fat meals.

Lack of time and energy almost certainly play a role, but
get this: Rose Frisch said Swedish researchers have proven

that fat gained in the bottom half of the body—remember, most pregnancy fat goes on the hips, thighs, and buttocks—really *is* biochemically different and harder to get rid of than fat in the face, abdomen, and other high places. Fat put on below the waist, said Frisch, simply doesn't break down for use as energy as easily as fat in the abdomen does—that is, unless you're pregnant or breastfeeding, in which case the body readily turns to fat below the waist for energy. (In fact, some experts believe that if you go into pregnancy already carrying saddlebags on your thighs, breastfeeding is the one and only opportunity you'll ever have—unless you opt for liposuction—to truly rid yourself of that particular fat.)

David V. Schapira, chief of the cancer prevention program at the H. Lee Moffitt Cancer Center & Research Institute at the University of South Florida, told the *Los Angeles Times* that according to his studies (mostly in the area of the relationship between abdominal fat and breast and endometrial cancers), fat cells in the upper body are larger and less numerous than cells in the buttocks and thighs. These fat cells in the abdomen have the greater potential for shrinkage, according to Schapira, while those in the lower body seem to be designed more for long-term storage.

Take comfort, however, if long past childbirth and breastfeeding you still possess stubborn, postpregnancy thunder thighs. Researchers have also found that fat stored in the bottom half of the body is nowhere near as dangerous as a "spare tire" around one's waist when it comes to heart disease risk. Why? "Apple-shaped" people tend to have higher cholesterol levels than "pear-shaped" people because their fat not only breaks down more easily but is stored much closer to the liver, and the liver responds to any fat that comes its way by producing more cholesterol.

Women who store fat below the belt are also at lower risk of developing diabetes and high blood pressure and of contracting breast and reproductive cancers than are apple-shaped women, according to Schapira and other researchers. This is believed to be because apple-shaped women produce more estrogen (see "Female Cancers" in this chapter).

Here's another bit of consolation if you're having trouble shedding "baby fat": you would be gaining weight even if you *didn't* have a baby. Obesity expert George Bray of the Pennington Biomedical Research Institute in New Orleans told *Health* magazine that "women will increase in weight as a result of hormones that prepare a woman's body for pregnancy—whether or not pregnancy occurs. I think about two pounds a decade is biologically appropriate."

In addition, metabolic rate (the rate at which we burn calories) slows down as we age, whether we have children or not. George Blackburn, M.D., associate professor of surgery at Harvard Medical School, told *Redbook* that for most people the metabolic rate is at its highest at age twenty-seven, then it starts slowing down about 3 percent every five years. "Between ages 27 and 47, your metabolic rate could decline as much as 12 percent," Blackburn said. What does this slowdown mean? That the body needs less energy to function. The example *Redbook* gave: If, at age 27, you need 1,800 calories a day to function, you'll need only 1,692 calories at age thirty-seven. But if you continue to eat 1,800 calories daily, the extra 108 calories will translate into one extra pound of body fat every thirty-three days.

Body Structure

Besides the revolutionary changes that occur in the pelvic area during pregnancy, your muscles, your ligaments, and occasionally even the bones that make up the rest of your body structure also undergo alteration that may be permanent.

The abdomen and rib cage. Thanks to the pregnancy hormone relaxin and the growth of the fetus, the ligaments and muscles in the abdominal area stretch out. The lowest three ribs on both sides of the rib cage also flare out to make room for the growing baby, and this is part of the reason the bra size of many pregnant women increases not just in cup size (e.g., from B to C) but also by back size (e.g., from a 34 to a 36).

Although the ligaments in the abdomen will "heal" to some extent after delivery, their chemical properties make them much less able to return to their prepregnancy state than muscles are, according to Doris Flood, a physical therapist with Kaiser Permanente in San Diego. Flood likens ligaments to rubber bands: you can stretch them out to capacity and they'll still have a little elasticity left to them, but they stay stretched out.

On the other hand, the abdominal muscles, which are stretched to twice their normal size by the time you deliver, can be returned almost to their prepregnancy condition—not, however, without exercise on your part. The consensus of the experts I consulted—OBs, fitness trainers, and physical therapists—was that the better toned your abdominal muscles were before pregnancy, the easier it is to get them back into shape postpartum. Getting your abdominal muscles back into shape after pregnancy not only flattens your tummy and whittles your waistline (the muscles are connected to those ribs that flared out, and exercise can help pull them back in), it may also remedy backaches because the abdominals play a major role in lower back support.

You can start a postpartum exercise program as soon as

your doctor gives the green light (usually at six weeks), and Chapter 3 contains suggestions about specific exercises and exercise programs. Anne Fehlman, who teaches pre- and postnatal exercise classes in southern California and is a personal fitness trainer specializing in new moms, said it takes about four to six months of regular exercise to get the abdominals back into prepregnancy shape. Fritzi Kallop, the nationally known childbirth educator, is less optimistic. She once told me that before she had her own children, she would blithely assure the women in her childbirth education classes that they'd have their waistlines back six to eight weeks after delivery. "I feel a little different about that since I had three large babies of my own," she told me. "If you are able to regain your prepregnant waistline before a year has passed, you are my true heroine!"

Recall that in the Introduction to this book I mentioned a mother whose doctor told her that even if she did eighteen hundred sit-ups a day her abdomen would never be as flat as it was prior to her pregnancy. The consensus among my experts: "After-baby abdominals will never again be as strong, and therefore they'll be more easily pushed out again—with another baby or a bowel problem, for example," said OB/GYN DiMarzo. "But those muscles can make your abdomen look every bit as flat as it used to be if you work at it."

Some women have not just slackened abdominal muscles but an additional problem called diastasis recti abdominis. This is a major tear of the band of connective tissue called the linea alba that runs down the median line of the abdominal wall and joins the abdominal muscles in the middle (it splits a little in all pregnant women). The significant tear usually occurs in women who were out of shape prepregnancy and who gain excessive weight during the pregnancy. Flood said the general rule of thumb among physical therapists is that if you can fit three fingers into this tear during or after pregnancy, the tear may cause significant problems for months postpartum. It can cause pain in the abdominal area, a downward displacement of the internal organs, and major back problems. "If you get diastasis recti abdominis during pregnancy, you're starting out postpartum in a very weakened state so it's easier to injure your back," Flood explained. In extreme cases, the separation may have to be corrected with surgery after the baby is born. Otherwise, physical therapists often help women minimize the problem by prescribing certain abdominal exercises in conjunction with an elasticized abdominal binder.

You can tell whether or not you are developing diastasis recti abdominis during pregnancy by lying on your back and bending your knees toward your chest. Next, by stretching your hands toward your feet, raise your shoulders and head slightly. Feel for the separation in the tissue in the middle of your abdomen near the belly button.

The spine. Some experts also believe that pregnancy can permanently change the curvature of the spine. Renata Shafor, M.D., a San Diego neurologist, once told me that a change in the curvature—which she says is caused by the pressure the fetus puts on the spine, particularly when a woman is lying on her back—may be to blame for an annoying malady called restless legs syndrome that is common in pregnancy. The syndrome makes pregnant women feel the need to move their legs constantly because they just can't seem to find a comfortable position for them, especially while lying down. Because the curvature change is permanent, some women continue to suffer a milder form of restless legs syndrome even after they've delivered (see Chapter 4 for more information).

The Postcesarean Body

Depending on how much labor was endured before surgery, women who have cesarean section generally do not have as much alteration in or damage to their vaginas or pelvic floors as women who deliver vaginally. "My gynecologist says I have the vagina of a sixteen-year-old," I once heard a three–C-section mother brag at a cocktail party (believe it or not).

With the uterus and abdominal wall, however, it's a different story, at least for the first few months after birth. The uterus and abdominal muscles were not only stretched but also cut, so they obviously need more healing time than those of the woman who delivered vaginally.

Cesarean incisions heal surprisingly fast, however, according to C-section expert Bruce Flamm, M.D., an OB/GYN with Kaiser Permanente in Riverside, California. They heal fast enough so that most women who have C-sections the first time and want to try a vaginal birth the second time will almost certainly be able to do so without any problems in as little as a year after the surgery. "All the healing that is going to be done will be done by then," said Flamm, who added that many doctors used to insist that their patients wait a lot longer between a C-section and a vaginal birth after cesarean (VBAC), if they permitted VBACs at all. In May 1993, Flamm released the results of a study of almost eleven thousand women who attempted vaginal birth after having had cesarean section(s). "We found that the risk of complications is very, very low," he said.

Flamm believes that after the uterine scar has healed (several weeks after surgery) there is no difference between the strength and condition of the uterus of a woman who had a C-section and her counterpart who delivered vaginally. This seems to be borne out by the statistics indicating that for the woman attempting a VBAC, the risk of uterine rupture—the reason so many mothers for so many years were told, "Once a cesarean, always a cesarean"—*is less than 1 percent.*

Even if a prior cesarean incision *does* rupture during a VBAC, it is apparently nowhere near as dangerous or even as dramatic as some doctors have lead some women to believe it would be. "I pictured a ruptured uterus to be like a bursting balloon, with a million little pieces flying throughout your body," one mother who eventually had a successful VBAC told me. According to Nancy Wainter Cohen and Lois J. Estner, who wrote a book called *Silent Knife,* "In the rare circumstances that a uterus with a previous cesarean does separate, the incision generally opens gently and neatly, like a seam or zipper." These authors go on to point out that the incidence of death in VBAC births is less for both the mother and infant than with elective repeat cesarean section.

In my research, I did come across one source—Mortimer Rosen, M.D., chairperson of the Department of Obstetrics and Gynecology at the College of Physicians and Surgeons at Columbia Presbyterian Hospital in New York City— who believes the younger siblings of a cesarean-delivered baby are at higher risk of having birth-related problems for another reason. "The placenta sticks to the wall of the uterus or bleeds more often in pregnancies following the cesarean, putting the younger sibling at greater risk," he wrote in his 1989 book, *The Cesarean Myth.*

Women who deliver by C-section are also at increased risk of secondary infertility (the inability to conceive a second child) because their surgery puts them at higher risk of developing postpartum infections in the reproductive tract, which can cause scarring and other problems associated with infertility.

Deborah Nemiro, M.D., a Scottsdale, Arizona, OB/ GYN, told me about one other not uncommon problem among women who have given birth via C-section: sometimes, because the surface of the healing uterine scar is raw, it adheres to the interior abdominal cavity wall and the uterus stays there instead of being free floating. Nemiro says that this problem doesn't have to be fixed, though it can sometimes cause pain and/or make the uterus feel larger and more prominent.

As for the abdominal scar, Nemiro says some women have trouble locating theirs a couple of years after surgery; at the other end of the spectrum, some women—particularly those who have had more than one C-section—will have a permanent "indentation," according to Nemiro.

I asked Bruce Flamm, can abdominal muscles that have been severed and then rejoined ever regain as much strength as muscles that have simply been stretched? "No studies have been done on that," he told me, "but my gut feeling [an apt choice of phrase, huh?] is that once those abdominal muscles are fully healed after a C-section, they're probably every bit as capable as those in the mother who delivered vaginally."

The Immune System

I asked Edwin Jacobson, M.D., a UCLA internist and nephrologist who has a special interest in chronic fatigue syndrome—which he believes is probably connected to an overactive immune system (see "Chronic Fatigue Syndrome" in this chapter)—if pregnancy and childbirth change the immune system in any long-lasting or permanent way. Specifically, I wanted to know whether mother-hood somehow makes us less immune to viruses and bacteria.

He said no, though he acknowledged that that may *seem* to be true. What's happening, he said, is that children, who have little immunity of their own, pick up, bring home, and expose us to scads of bugs. "Living with a toddler is like a constant viral hurricane," Jacobson said.

In terms of colds alone, the average young child gets three to eight a year, and the parents typically catch about half of those. "The year my little girl entered preschool, the three of us got five colds plus three other viruses that made us barf," one mom told me. "That was the first time I'd thrown up in sixteen years."

I later found out that most of us are swooped up by the viral hurricane long before our babies enter toddlerhood. One of the most intriguing aspects of the 1989 postpartum study of 436 first-time mothers in St. Paul was how common respiratory illnesses were in these women. The percentage of women with at least one respiratory symptom—such as a cough or a stuffed-up nose—rose from 25 percent at one month postpartum to a whopping 42 percent at three months, then remained greater than 40 percent for the rest of the first year. Women who went back to work during the first year had more respiratory infections than those who didn't, and the researchers believe that's probably due to several factors—including the infant's exposure to infections at day care, the mother's exposure to the illnesses of coworkers, and the mother's increased susceptibility to infection because of work stress. Stress—proven in many studies to be an immune system suppressor—is probably the primary reason that all mothers get sick so often in that tough first year.

Migraines and Other Maladies

Migraines. One of the biggest postpregnancy body changes for me was that the number of migraine headaches I suffer in a typical month increased from about one to three and sometimes four. When I first started to study pregnancy's long-term and permanent changes to the body, I asked a doctor about this. He told me I couldn't pin the blame for the increased headaches on pregnancy itself. He suggested that I was probably getting more headaches simply because now that I had a child I was under more stress than I had been prebaby.

My mistake was in asking an OB/GYN about this instead of a neurologist. He was confusing tension headaches, caused by strain on facial, neck, and scalp muscles, with migraine headaches (sometimes called vascular headaches), which are caused by swelling blood vessels in the head that result in strain within their walls. I did not argue with his theory despite my understanding that you do not wake up in the morning with a *tension* headache.

Eventually, I did ask a neurologist about this. Stephen Silberstein, M.D., a neurologist at Germantown Hospital and Medical Center in Philadelphia, told me that many women who are prone to migraine (a whopping 18 percent of all women) do see an increase in these attacks after becoming mothers and that *the increase can indeed be traced to the pregnancy*. In fact, some women (about 11 percent) get their *first* migraine while they're pregnant. Silberstein said the trigger is pregnancy's high estrogen levels. He is a believer in the theory that pregnancy permanently alters a woman's hormonal levels, which explains why some women see an increase in migraine attacks for years after pregnancy. "It's almost as if you set the process in motion during the pregnancy and then every month after is like a minipregnancy, with the estrogen levels rising and falling, triggering migraine," Silberstein said.

Interestingly, migraine sufferers usually get a six-month vacation (the second and third trimesters) from migraines during pregnancy, according to Silberstein. He says "migrainers"—as neurologists refer to us—usually have one or more attacks in the first trimester, when hormones are raging, then see months of relief after the hormones stabilize and remain stable until childbirth. Silberstein cited study statistics that confirm this: of 703 pregnant women, 116 had migraine headaches during pregnancy. Of those with migraines, 100 had had migraines before they got pregnant; 16 got their first migraines while pregnant. Of the 116, 70 percent saw improvement in their second and third trimesters.

Endometriosis. In the common condition called endometriosis, the tissues of the endometrium (the lining of the uterus) spread to and begin to grow on the organs outside the uterus instead of being expelled through the vagina each month during menstruation. Typical symptoms include extreme menstrual cramps, abdominal pain, and painful intercourse. Because the endometrial tissue adheres to the ovaries and fallopian tubes, the disease is also a frequent cause of infertility; it can interfere with the release of the egg from the ovary or with the egg's journey down the fallopian tube.

The good news about the frustrating malady is that, because endometriosis is related to menstruation, its progress is halted during pregnancy and breastfeeding because you're not menstruating. Pregnancy and breastfeeding also give you a vacation from the pain endometriosis usually causes during menstruation.

More good news: if you have endometriosis, are treated

for it, and then have a baby, your chances of getting the disease back again are lower than if you simply get treated for it and don't have a baby, according to gynecologist Neysa Whiteman. Why? Whiteman said experts don't know yet. "I think that pregnancy just burns it all out," she said. "Pregnancy just seems to make endometriosis go away more completely than it does when you use drugs and other interventions to treat it."

Whiteman showed me a heartening study conducted by the Department of Obstetrics and Gynecology at Cornell Medical College. Of sixty-eight previously infertile women with endometriosis who had been treated with surgery or drugs and then went on to deliver a child, fifty-two of them were able to conceive a second child, twenty-eight within a year. In showing me this study, Whiteman stressed that pregnancy is not a guarantee that endometriosis will never return. She said that many women in the study probably conceived their second babies before endometriosis even had a *chance* to return. "Still, pregnancy seems to be a permanent solution in many cases," she said.

Pregnancy has also long been considered an excellent way to prevent endometriosis in the first place. Women who start their childbearing early and then have several babies rarely get this malady. Their reproductive organs simply never have enough time to get the endometriosis process up and going. According to the medical reference work *Kistner's Gynecology*, the typical woman with endometriosis has had "uninterrupted cyclic menstruation" for five or more years.

Okay, so what if you have one baby at eighteen and that's it? Can't you go on to develop endometriosis at twenty-five or thirty-five? Whiteman says it's possible but not very likely, not in her experience. Why? To date, this is another medical mystery. But don't you love it?

Premenstrual syndrome (PMS). If you suffer from premenstrual syndrome, you get relief during pregnancy. This is because the fluctuating hormonal levels of the menstrual cycle cease when there's no menstruation, and these fluctuating levels are believed by most—but not all—experts to be somehow responsible for PMS (at this point, no one is exactly sure how). (See "PMS Busters" in Chapter 3 for more theories.)

Physician Nancy Cetel, one of the authors of the 1984 study that proved once and for all that PMS is a verifiable medical condition, told me that whether and how PMS returns after pregnancy is variable. Some women never get it back again or have much milder symptoms. "As a rule, however, women suffer more from PMS as they get older and have more children," Cetel said.

In fact, according to Whiteman, most women with PMS complain that they never had it until after they gave birth (or, interestingly, until after they stopped taking the birth control pill). That's also been the observation of Katharina Dalton, the British physician considered to be the world's foremost expert on PMS. In her book *Once a Month*, she said PMS symptoms such as irritability take many mothers by surprise. "They find themselves becoming quick-tempered and making totally irrational decisions," she said. "They become impatient with the children, not waiting for them to learn to dress or eat for themselves. They become intolerant, won't accept that 'kids will be kids,' shout at them when they are playing harmlessly, and complain that the children won't behave."

Cetel, Dalton, and Whiteman all agree that after children come into your life, environmental circumstances (such as more stress, less sleep) may exacerbate PMS symptoms. But they also agree that there's an internal force at work. Dalton's theory is that the onset of PMS after pregnancy—or the worsening of its symptoms—has something to do with the fact that pregnancy is a time when the menstruation controlling center in the hypothalamus area of the brain has been upset. (Other times this happens: puberty, stopping the pill, being sterilized, or having a hysterectomy.)

Along those lines, Cetel said, "One as yet unproven but interesting theory is that pregnancy causes lasting hormonal changes that make the body more susceptible to PMS." This seems to jibe with the school of thought I first mentioned in the section about migraine headaches: that once you have a baby, every menstrual cycle is like a minipregnancy. I talked to several women who get PMS symptoms that they never had until they were pregnant. One woman, for example, told me that in the few days before her period begins, she is very sensitive to and put off by the same odors that made her sick in the first trimester of pregnancy: green onions, barbecuing meat, and the smell of a fireplace the morning after there was a fire in it. (See "PMS Busters" in Chapter 3 for some suggestions on coping with this condition.)

Asthma and other allergies. Two moms I know of had allergies that either began or got worse after pregnancy. Anita developed an allergy to laundry detergent after the birth of her third child, and my own hay fever suddenly took a permanent turn for the worse, requiring prescription medication, shortly after I had Madeline.

John Winder, M.D., a practicing allergist in Toledo, Ohio, a Fellow of the American College of Allergy and Immunology, and a frequent spokesman for that organization, told me that although he's heard several anecdotes like mine and Anita's, he knows of no studies on the topic of whether pregnancy and childbirth cause antibody levels—which are tied to allergies—"to go from X to Y or stay the same or whatever," as he put it. He said that it's possible that pregnancy can alter antibody levels, but he stressed that it's more likely that the allergic reactions Anita and I suffered are linked to environmental factors rather than pregnancy. Winder said, for example, that Anita may have been sensitive to detergent all along but perhaps didn't have enough exposure to it to cause a reaction until the laundry load increase that accompanied her third child.

As for my hay fever, Winder speculated that it got worse because I began spending more time around my house, which is in a heavily vegetated, semirural area, after Madeline was born. I started to argue with him, to tell him that I worked at home *before* she was born, too. But then it occurred to me that in my premotherhood days, I did spend many afternoons doing research in the library or interviewing experts at their places of business in person. Nowadays, I do most of my research and interviewing via phone and computer. At home.

The one allergy-related condition allergists have studied extensively in regard to pregnancy's effect on it is asthma, the condition in which the bronchi (the main air passages of the lungs) become partially obstructed because the muscles in the bronchial walls contract. Most asthma is triggered by an allergy, such as to eggs or pollen. "About one-third of women with asthma will get worse during pregnancy, one-third will get better, and one-third will stay the same," said Winder.

Will women whose asthma gets better during pregnancy stay better after pregnancy? "Not necessarily," said Winder. "It will often go back to the way it was prepregnancy. But it's just not predictable." What *is* predictable, he said, is that whatever happens to your asthma in your first pregnancy will most likely reoccur in your subsequent pregnancies.

Winder said that the changes in asthma during pregnancy are due to high hormonal levels and fluid changes that occur in the body. He said the effect of the growing fetus on breathing capacity also plays a role, but that if there's going to be a change in asthma, it will occur in the first trimester, when the tiny fetus is obviously having its least effect on breathing capacity.

He added that, while there have been no formal studies, he has heard of isolated cases of women who developed asthma for the first time during pregnancy. "That doesn't mean the asthma wasn't there before pregnancy; it may be that it just wasn't of such a degree that the women noticed it," Winder said. He agreed, however, that pregnancy's revolutionary effects on the body could conceivably bring on asthma in the first place.

Winder discussed one other pregnancy-related condition worth noting. He said he's examined many mothers, toting babies or even toddlers, who complain that their noses became plugged while they were pregnant and have remained that way long past birth. Winder said that what happened to these women started out as a condition called vasomotor rhinitis of pregnancy. Because the erectile tissues throughout the body become more sensitive to hormones during pregnancy, the lining of some women's noses swells up in the first few weeks of the first trimester, causing severe nasal congestion. Winder said this condition resolves itself within weeks. But in an effort to relieve the congestion without taking pills, some women (such as the mothers mentioned above) resort to a nasal decongestant spray—and their noses literally become addicted to it. Because of the chemicals in such a spray, if you use it more than about three days in a row, it begins to have a rebound effect: your nose clears up right after you use the spray; then, as the spray wears off, the nose congests even a little bit more than before. "The more you use it, the less effective it becomes," said Winder, "to the point where you're using a bottle of spray a week, spraying six, eight, or ten times a day—instead of twice in twenty-four hours, as the label suggests—just to keep the nose minimally open."

Winder said pregnant women with vasomotor rhinitis should ask their obstetricians if they may take an oral decongestant, such as Sudafed, that does not have the spray's rebound effect. He also recommended the use of a nonchemical saltwater nasal spray (there are many brands available over the counter). Winder said exercise is another natural way of unplugging the nose. "It's a normal physiological response when you exercise that the nasal membranes shrink down to give you better airflow into the nose," he said.

Gallstones. One of the biggest after-baby shocks to my friend and fellow writer Lisa was a gallstone. About four weeks after she gave birth in early 1993, she had to go to a hospital emergency room late one night "in as much pain as I was during labor," she said. After the emergency room doctor diagnosed a gallstone, he told her that these stones are a common side effect of pregnancy.

Though gallstones—which range in size from a pinhead to a chicken egg—can dissolve on their own, in many cases they can cause pain and digestive problems and often require surgery, as did the one in Lisa's case. Gallstones are created in the gallbladder, which is connected to the liver and the small intestine by two tubes. The gallbladder holds up to a cup of what's called bile, a substance needed to break down fat and assist the body in absorbing it. Bile is made up of cholesterol, bile acids, and electrolytes, and gallstones form when there is too much cholesterol and too little bile acid. The cholesterol becomes so thick that it crystallizes into stones and obstructs the bile flow. Ouch, as Lisa learned.

I asked James Everhart, M.D., of the National Institute of Diabetes and Digestive Disorders, why pregnant women are especially susceptible to gallstones. He said that for one thing, thanks to elevated estrogen levels during pregnancy, the cholesterol in the bile increases and gets thicker. The second reason he believes pregnant women are at increased risk of gallstones is that the elevated levels of progesterone in the body decrease the efficiency of the gallbladder; it does not contract as well, so it does not send the bile to the small intestine as efficiently. As a result, there's more of it to sit around in the gallbladder and get concentrated and form gallstones.

Just how common is the problem in pregnant women and new mothers? Everhart told me about a very recent study conducted at Catholic University in Santiago, Chile. Researchers used noninvasive sonography to look at the gallbladders of women who had given birth just two or three days earlier and women who had never given birth. They found gallstones in 12.2 percent of the mothers, compared to only 1.3 percent of the women who had never given birth. Of that 12.2 percent, 31 percent had gallstone symptoms (mostly abdominal pain). In one-fourth of the women with gallstones, the stones eventually disappeared on their own.

Here's the good news: when researchers took a second look at the gallbladders of the mothers—this time a couple of months after birth—they "did not have bile that would suggest the development of gallstones," according to Everhart. Apparently, once your hormone levels return to normal after pregnancy and breastfeeding, so does your gallbladder. Everhart believes, however, that women who had gallstones in their first pregnancies are at much higher risk of developing them again in subsequent pregnancies.

He added that obesity is another risk factor when it comes to gallstones. This is probably because women with a lot of body fat have more estrogen circulating in their bodies, and estrogen increases the amount and thickness of cholesterol in the bile. Therefore, if a woman is both pregnant and overweight, she is at especially high risk for developing gallstones.

Carpal tunnel syndrome and other hand problems. One of the more unusual findings of the 1989 St. Paul study of women in their first postpartum year was that many suffered numbness and tingling in their hands. According to Patricia Jenkyns, a physical therapist at the Maternal and Child Health Center at Cambridge Physical Therapy in Cambridge, Massachusetts, some of these women probably were suffering from carpal tunnel syndrome, a painful condition in which a major nerve that carries signals between the brain and the hand becomes severely pinched when surrounding tissues are swollen. Jenkyns said pregnancy is a prime time for this condition to begin, since the extra fluids circulating in the body can and usually do cause swelling. She said that as the fluids in the body decrease after childbirth, carpal tunnel syndrome often resolves itself, but it's a slow process.

Some women find relief by wearing a brace or splint on the wrist. Other treatments include a physician-prescribed diuretic or steroid injection to combat the inflammation. Sometimes only surgery that creates more space around the nerve alleviates the problem. Fortunately, this is a fairly simple operation that requires only a brief hospital stay and leaves just the hint of a scar.

Another postpartum problem that can cause pain, numbness, and tingling in the wrists and hands, according to Jenkyns, is tendinitis of the thumbs. Though this is often misdiagnosed as carpal tunnel syndrome, it is an *overuse* syndrome, Jenkyns said, caused by repeated lifting and carrying of the baby. One friend who was diagnosed with this problem got the same treatment she would have had for carpal tunnel syndrome—a brace plus shots to lessen the inflammation. Jenkyns said physical therapists start with "rest and ice" to cure the problem. "Sometimes we use ultrasound or friction massage to quiet the tendinitis," she said, "but finally you have to learn to lift the baby without using your thumbs to decrease stress to the area."

Finally, Jenkyns said postpartum hand and finger problems might also be the result of what's called thoracic outlet syndrome, which often occurs in combination with one of the problems discussed above. Thoracic outlet syndrome is a compression of the brachial plexus—all of the vessels and nerves that go to your hands—in the armpit or right in front of the shoulder. This often starts in pregnancy as the increasing heaviness of the breasts and uterus pull a woman into a forward bend; that bending continues after birth as she cares for her baby. In this case, Jenkyns said, the cure is changing postural habits—bringing the shoulders back and strengthening the upper back muscles.

Osteoporosis. Since the 1940s, many in the medical community believed that the risk of osteoporosis (the thinning-bones condition common in postmenopausal women) increased with the number of children a woman bore and the spacing of those births. The theory was that frequent pregnancies caused more calcium to be "borrowed" from the bone than could be "repaid" by the diet. This theory has been disproven. Researchers at the University of California at San Diego released a study in late 1992 showing that there is no significant association between bone density and either the number of pregnancies or breastfeeding history when age or obesity are taken into account. One of the reasons for this finding is that, in the United States at least, the diets of pregnant women are nutritionally sound enough so that the fetus's calcium requirement can be fulfilled strictly from the mother's ingestion of food.

Diabetes. In diabetes, a metabolic disorder, the body does not make or use insulin properly. Many women first get diabetes during pregnancy. Gestational diabetes mellitus (GDM), as this form of the disorder is known, occurs when a pregnant woman's pancreas is unable to make enough insulin to counter the rise in her blood sugar caused by the higher amounts of hormones in her body.

GDM differs from the other types of diabetes (Type I and Type II) in that it is not usually permanent, said Sunita C. Baxi, M.D., an endocrinologist and coordinator of the team that cares for pregnant women at the Whittier Institute for Diabetes and Endocrinology in La Jolla, California. However, a small percentage of women with GDM, according to Baxi, do go on to develop Type II diabetes later in life, especially those who remain overweight and/or have a family history of the disorder. GDM can reoccur in subsequent pregnancies; the risk is higher than for someone who didn't have it the first time. For this reason, Baxi said women who have had GDM in the past should be screened for it sometime between the sixteenth and twentieth weeks of the new pregnancy rather than between twenty-four and twenty-eight weeks, which is standard for all pregnant women.

According to Baxi, women who are already diabetic when they become pregnant are in for some changes, too.

She said that the insulin requirement for women with Type I diabetes increases as the pregnancy progresses. That's also true for women with Type II diabetes, who are generally taken off oral medication and placed on insulin for the duration of the pregnancy. Baxi said that in both cases insulin requirements drop to prepregnancy levels after the baby is born. In other words, pregnancy and childbirth generally have no lasting effect on diabetes—unless, said gynecologist Neysa Whiteman, the diabetes is not properly controlled during pregnancy. Then it can worsen existing eye or renal (kidney) problems.

AIDS. Because data about women and AIDS were scarce in the early years of the AIDS epidemic, experts apparently relied solely on anecdotal information and declared that it was dangerous for an HIV-positive woman to get pregnant, because the pregnancy would speed up the course of the disease. Since then, however, pregnancy studies all over the world have revealed that pregnancy has very little or no impact on the course of the disease in women.

The chance of passing HIV on to the baby just before birth or just after birth is also much less than originally feared. Generally, transmission of HIV occurs in 25 percent of children born to HIV-infected women.

On the other hand, researchers are finding that a woman who is HIV positive may be at more risk of infecting her partner when she is pregnant than when she's not. Women typically have an increase in cervical mucus during pregnancy, and that mucus may in turn have an increased number of HIV-containing cells.

Chronic fatigue syndrome (CFS). The mysterious debilitating ailment that is known as chronic fatigue syndrome produces symptoms such as fever and swollen glands and leaves sufferers feeling weak, bone-tired, achy, and frequently depressed for months or even years at a time. "Nobody knows exactly what causes it, but we're all pretty convinced that sufferers have overactive immune systems," said Edwin Jacobson, who has seen hundreds of CFS patients. He said that no formal studies have been done—he's trying to get funding for one—but in the experience of UCLA doctors, women with CFS *get better* when they're pregnant, and the old symptoms usually don't come back after the baby is born. Jacobson and his colleagues have no idea at this point why this is so. "It may be due to hormonal changes, psychological changes, or both," he said.

Heart disease. University of Pennsylvania researchers announced in mid-1993 that women who have been pregnant at least six times are more prone to experiencing a heart attack or some form of heart disease than other women are. Using data from the Framington Heart Study of five thousand women, researchers found that women with half a dozen pregnancies had a 70 percent higher heart disease risk than women who had never been pregnant. Women with "multiple pregnancies of five or less" had a 30 percent higher risk. So far, these findings appear to be purely statistical; I haven't found any speculation on what factors lie behind the numbers. Could it be that multiple pregnancies are taxing on the heart? Or is it the stress of rearing six kids? More research is definitely in order.

Female Cancers

This section is brimming with good news for mothers.

Breast cancer. Having a baby appears to decrease your risk of contracting breast cancer (with one exception that we'll get to in a minute). According to breast surgeon Sheryl Cramer, most breast cancers are linked to estrogen. Therefore, the longer you're exposed to estrogen, the greater your risks. When we're not pregnant, our bodies get a virtual estrogen bath every month in order to ensure we go through the whole ovulation/menstruation cycle. This is not the case while we're pregnant. During pregnancy, estrogen continues to circulate in the body. But of the three types of estrogen produced during pregnancy, the one that increases the most is estriol, which doesn't bind well to the breast, according to Brian E. Henderson, M.D., director of the Kenneth Norris, Jr. Comprehensive Cancer Center at the University of Southern California. Also, according to Cramer, estrogen's effects are counteracted during pregnancy by high levels of the other pregnancy hormones, such as progesterone and prolactin. These conditions also exist during the breastfeeding period, Cramer said, so if you nurse you prolong the period you're protected from estrogen's negative effects.

But after childbirth and nursing, it's cycle time again. Even if we have one or two children, most of us will ovulate about 450 times in our lifetimes. Experts are pointing to that astounding number as one big reason breast cancer rates have surged in the last few decades. In comparison, breast cancer was virtually unknown among our ancestors two hundred years ago. Why? Because they didn't begin menstruating till they were about seventeen (compared to our average age of twelve), they started having babies right after that, and they gave birth to an average of eight children apiece, so they typically had only 150 ovulations in their lifetimes.

Having a baby decreases your risk of getting breast cancer for another reason besides the estrogen vacation. Recall reading earlier in this chapter about the massive permanent changes in the breasts that pregnancy, birth, and breastfeeding are responsible for. These changes in effect "set" the breast cells and make them much more resistant to genetic mutations such as cancer. It stands to reason, then, that the more cyclical estrogen a breast is exposed to before it undergoes this "maturity," as some researchers refer to it, the greater the risk of cancer. A woman who has her first child at age eighteen has only a third the cancer risk of the first-time mother who's forty.

This seemed pretty logical to me. Why then, I wondered as I did my initial research, did I keep coming across data indicating that a woman who delays having her first baby until after age thirty has a *higher* risk of contracting breast cancer than a woman who *never* has children? I took this complaint to Mitchell H. Gail, M.D., a biostatistician at the National Cancer Institute, who himself had published statistics in support of that anomaly.

"My work has been more descriptive than explanatory," Gail told me. "What we've tried to do here is summarize what the data are telling us rather than interpret it." He did say, however, that the difference in risk was relatively small when compared to other risk factors. And he also said that there appears to be another factor (a genetic one) in this no kids versus kids after thirty risk factor comparison. "From our data, it appears that if you have no children and happen to be from a family in which no close relatives have been affected by breast cancer, your risk is somewhat lower than that of a woman in the same situation but who had children after age thirty," Gail said. "Things change around if you have a strong family history—let's say two or more affected relatives. Then the woman without children is at slightly higher risk than the woman who had children after age thirty. So it's not absolutely clear-cut."

Cramer backed him up: "It's very confusing, and those

particular risk factors are relatively insignificant. Reproductive history, age [at first childbirth], and family history *together* account for only 25 percent of breast-cancer cases. Those factors just tend to get played up because they're among the few you actually have some control over. Psychologically, all of us want to feel we have some control. When I address women's groups about breast cancer, I am always asked, 'What can I do to lower my risks?' And all I can say is 'Choose your grandparents carefully.' That's by far the most important thing you can do!"

There's some interesting new information, however, about how you might be able to decrease your daughter's risk of later contracting breast cancer. Researchers have found that the amount of estrogen circulating in a mother's body while she's pregnant may have some impact on a female fetus's future cancer risks. Again, this is a case of the less estrogen the better, and apparently you can have some control over this by being careful about your pregnancy weight gain. A baby who weighs more than eight pounds is considered at higher risk for future breast cancer because her mother may have put on more fat than the mother of a smaller baby, and fat has been linked to higher estrogen levels. The babies of mothers who have toxemia— a disorder of late pregnancy characterized by high blood pressure—are considered at lower risk because that condition typically signifies lower estrogen levels.

Ovarian cancer. The risk of contracting ovarian cancer, like that of breast cancer, is strongly related to a woman's relative exposure to estrogen and the number of ovulations she has. That's why your risk for this cancer, too, is less (some 30 to 60 percent less) if you have given birth to a child or—even better—children. A spokesperson for the Gilda Radner Familial Ovarian Cancer Registry, which is affiliated with the Roswell Park Cancer Institute in Buffalo, New York, told me that pregnancy "shuts the ovaries down and gives them a rest."

It stops the process by which, each month, small cysts form on or near the ovary as a normal part of ovulation. Usually, these cysts pop and disappear within days. Sometimes, however, they can last into the next cycle or cycles if your hormones are unbalanced, if you're under stress, or for other reasons. If such a cyst sits there long enough, "it has the potential for turning bad," as the registry spokesperson put it. "And we believe that ovarian cancer may start in one of these cysts that has gone bad."

She went on to say that having your first child after the age of thirty does increase your ovarian cancer risk; why this is so with *breast* cancer has been explained somewhat, but no one has yet answered that question in regard to ovarian cancer. Researchers are working on it. According to the registry, however, if you have a first baby after thirty or even forty, your ovarian cancer risk is still lower than that of someone who never gave birth at all.

Uterine cancer. Uterine cancer is also linked to estrogen exposure, according to the National Cancer Institute. Women who take estrogen or have estrogen replacement therapy after menopause are especially at risk for this form of cancer. As with both breast and ovarian cancer, your risk of contracting uterine cancer decreases with each child you bear, since pregnancy and, to a lesser extent, breast-feeding, give you a vacation from the estrogen-rich process of ovulation. But here's one refreshing difference: according to the National Cancer Institute, a woman who bears her last child after age thirty-four has a lower uterine cancer risk than a woman who completes her family at a younger age. Researchers aren't sure yet why this is so.

Endometrial and cervical cancer. While women who have given birth have a lower risk of contracting endometrial cancer (cancer in the lining of the uterus) for many of the same reasons discussed above, a spokesperson for the National Cancer Institute told me that, as far as we know right now, there doesn't seem to be any tie between reproductive history and *cervical* cancer risk. The latest research available indicates that the primary risk factors for cancer of the cervix are smoking, number of sex partners, and exposure to the papilloma virus (genital warts).

Other Forms of Cancer

More good, and somewhat surprising, news: women who have given birth seem to have a significantly lower risk of contracting bladder, colon, and especially brain cancer. According to Kenneth P. Cantor, M.D., an epidemiologist with the National Cancer Institute, various recent studies (including some of his own) indicate that mothers have only 40 percent of the risk for brain cancer that nonmothers do and only 60 percent of the risk for bladder and colon cancer.

I was amazed that childbirth could have any sort of influence on the risk of getting cancer in organs that are not involved in the reproductive process. I pressed Cantor for an explanation, and he said, "The idea is that there are hormone receptors on the surface of these [cancer] cells that would influence cell proliferation."

You mean, I said, that, as is the case with many breast and ovarian cancers, these other cancers are bred or fed by hormones and that during pregnancy and breastfeeding you're suppressing those hormones? He responded, "We don't know yet. I'm just going to plead ignorance."

But doesn't that sound logical? I think so.

Cantor told me that in the dozen or so studies done on

colon cancer and reproductive history, the number of children one has borne seems to have more influence on risk than one's age at the first birth does. As for bladder and brain cancer, Cantor himself conducted a large study that included these types of cancers, and he said that, other than the general finding that mothers have less relative risk than nonmothers, no one knows the specifics yet, such as whether the number of children you bear has anything to do with it. In a paper he wrote about the bladder cancer portion of the study, however, he did note that he saw a trend—though he called it a "statistically insignificant trend"—suggestive of a decreasing bladder cancer risk with *increasing* [my italics] age at first birth." The reason Cantor and his associates who conducted the brain and bladder cancer studies don't know more of the specifics is that they weren't even looking at reproductive history as a risk factor; they were studying other risk factors. They asked the women who participated very few questions about their reproductive histories. "But when we saw the differences in risks between mothers and nonmothers, we thought it was extremely important to publish these findings so that other people will conduct studies, using our work as a serious hypothesis," Cantor said. "Just keep in mind that our findings are very preliminary, and much more study is needed."

Cantor said he and his colleagues looked at rectal, kidney, and pancreatic cancers in the same study as the brain and bladder cancers and found no association between rectal and pancreatic cancers and motherhood or nonmotherhood. With kidney cancer, women who had given birth were at slightly higher risk than women who had not. Cantor said, however, that the numbers in this case were "statistically unstable," which means we shouldn't take this finding too seriously.

Even if you place a kidney cancer risk in the "negatives" column, don't forget that motherhood *reduces* your cancer risks in so many other cases: breast, ovarian, endometrial, uterine, brain, bladder, and colon. Decreasing your cancer risk is truly one of the most wonderful ways having a baby changes your body forever.

Pain

Doctors have long conceded that females are better at enduring pain than males. This is pretty impressive, since we are also more tactilely sensitive than males, meaning we feel pain more acutely. The theory is that Mother Nature gave us greater fortitude in the face of pain because we must go through so much of it in order to bear children and continue the species.

Evidently, females who have given birth show even more resilience to pain than nonmothers do, at least according to one expert. Physical therapist Doris Flood, who deals with people in pain all day long, said almost all of her female patients who are being treated for pain are *not mothers*. Why? Flood and I can only speculate. Maybe we just don't have time to focus on or deal with pain. Or maybe the experience of labor and delivery "which goes so far beyond pain that the word doesn't adequately describe it," as one friend put it, just makes us more tolerant of lesser aches and pains.

Strength and Fitness Level

Let's bring this chapter to a close on a real upper.

Not a lot of studies have been done on this, but evidence is mounting that you can actually *improve* your cardiovascular fitness while you're pregnant. Explains the Melpomene Institute for Women's Health Research in the book *The Bodywise Woman*: "Your oxygen consumption—a measure of fitness that is also called aerobic capacity—increases throughout your term until it is 30 percent greater than the nonpregnant level. Studies indicate that you can actually increase your aerobic capacity by exercising while you are pregnant."

Pregnancy also may affect a woman's strength. Several mothers have told me that they are physically stronger than they were before they had a baby. But this raises a "which came first, the chicken or the egg" question: are these women stronger because of some lasting effect pregnancy has on the body or because they've built up muscles by hoisting a baby/toddler/preschooler in and out of a crib/car seat/high chair/bathtub a thousand times a day? It's probably both. Carol Ann Weber, a Marina del Rey, California-based bodybuilder who writes and speaks frequently on that topic, is one of several firm believers that you have a unique opportunity during pregnancy to increase your strength. She told me that several prominent competitive female bodybuilders reported an increase in strength while weight training during pregnancy. While all of these women experienced a subsequent decrease in that training strength after they gave birth (usually to their original strength level, or even lower), they all reported a postpartum *increase* in their endurance levels, according to Weber. And, said Weber, after their hormonal levels returned to normal sometime in the first postpartum year, the women reported that they not only regained their original training strength but that it became better than *ever*. In fact, Weber said many bodybuilders get increasingly stronger with each subsequent baby.

In her book *Pregnancy and Sports Fitness*, sports physician and bodybuilder Lynne Pirie devoted several pages to

runners who, sometimes only a few months after childbirth, came back to better their prepregnancy records.
Marathoner Miki Gorman, for example, ran a world best
time in 1973 of 2:46:36. She had a baby in early 1975 and
then, at age 41, won the New York City Marathon in 1976,
improving on her record by seven minutes. Pirie noted that
there were rumors in the past that pre-1991 "Soviet"
Russian and other Eastern European coaches, aware of
pregnancy's apparent benefits on performance and training capacity, advised their top women competitors to give
birth two years before the Olympic Games.

Closer to home is the postpartum experience of my
friend Kim, an avid runner and the mother of a one-year-
old. "I have more stamina now than I've ever had," she
said.

What's going on here? Weber has researched the question of why strength can be gained during pregnancy, and
she believes the production of certain hormones and the
increased levels of others can increase muscle strength and
promote muscle growth. In *Pregnancy and Sports Fitness*,
Lynne Pirie said that doctors, coaches, and athletes can't
explain why performance improves in many cases after
pregnancy. Then she tossed out several hypotheses: "Could
it be that pregnant women are unintentionally training
while carrying around a 25-pound handicap? Do they
develop *other* muscles as they carry their baby? Will these
beneficial results last, and if so, how long after a pregnancy? Is it possible a woman who has a baby, after having
already proved herself as an athlete, wants to show the
world she is *still* an athlete of championship quality?"

Another source I checked, the book *Modern Principles of
Athletic Training*, by two Cal State Long Beach professors
of physical education, agreed that many female athletes
perform better after childbirth. The authors speculated

that this may be because the hormonal system has been permanently and advantageously altered. In their more technical terms: "It has been postulated that pregnancy and childbirth activate latent endocrinological forces that manifest themselves in an improved physical efficiency."

I shouted this explanation out my office window when Kim jogged by one day. "Why ask why?" she shouted back. "All I know is that I love it."

Appendix A at the end of this book provides a quick reference of body changes we have explored in this chapter. It summarizes, alphabetically by body part and condition/disease, the long-term and permanent physical changes you can expect after childbirth.

CHAPTER THREE

TAKING CARE
OF YOUR
POSTBABY BODY

You can do a lot of things to make yourself feel better and to speed up your progress toward a new and improved you. Let's start with those first revolutionary weeks.

Coping with Physical Transitions

Afterpains. Postpartum uterine contractions stop even before most first-time mothers leave the hospital. But if yours don't and they're really bothering you at home, try putting a heating pad on your abdomen or—what works even better—take a couple of ibuprofen tablets (but get your doctor's okay first). Ibuprofen—Nuprin and Advil are popular brands—works as well on afterpains as it does on menstrual cramps.

Episiotomy. The usual causes of discomfort at the site of your episiotomy are swelling, dried-out stitches, and the accumulation of vaginal fluids in the stitches. Swelling should be a problem only in the first few postpartum days.

To ease the discomfort of swelling, most doctors recommend wearing an ice pack for the first twenty-four hours and then taking warm sitz baths (in which you use only a couple of inches of water) after that. But William Droegemueller, M.D., who chairs the departments of obstetrics and gynecology at the University of North Carolina, told *American Baby* magazine that he disagrees with the warm sitz baths part of this standard regimen. He thinks a new mother with an episiotomy should take *ice-cold* sitz baths because ice reduces swelling, muscle irritability, and spasm in *any* kind of injury (for athletic injuries, he points out, ice baths have replaced hot whirlpool baths). He recommends filling the tub with a couple of inches of cold tap water and then adding as much ice as you can stand and staying in for twenty to thirty minutes.

You should take whichever kind of sitz bath—warm or cold—makes you feel better. Many hospitals supply new mothers with a portable sitz bath that fits over the toilet seat.

Some of the moms I talked to preferred wearing ice packs at home to taking sitz baths, and they made reasonable facsimiles of the kind you get in the hospital by filling plastic bags with crushed ice. One enterprising mom, out of ice and desperate, substituted a small bag of frozen peas and was delighted with the result: "They hold their cold better than ice," she reported. A bag of frozen popcorn kernels (not the microwave variety) supposedly works even better.

Between ice packs and/or sitz baths, you may want to use an anesthetic spray or ointment (ask your doctor or a nurse for recommendations). A lot of women I interviewed swore by Tucks pads or a generic equivalent, gauze pads dipped in refrigerated witch hazel. These things soothe both soreness and itching.

One important way to lessen discomfort and prevent problems in the healing perineal area is to keep it clean. Change your sanitary pads often and use the "peri" bottle the hospital will probably give you to squirt the incision area when you shower. You may also want to do this every time you go to the bathroom. Always wipe from front to back when you have a bowel movement to prevent the episiotomy area from becoming contaminated with feces.

Incidentally, some experts believe you can speed up the healing of an episiotomy by doing Kegels (see "Tighten Up: K Power!" in this chapter). These exercises are believed to help pull the stitches together.

Hemorrhoids. Much of what makes an episiotomy feel better makes hemorrhoids less uncomfortable, too. Try a sitz bath, for example. Here again experts can't seem to agree on whether a shallow cool bath or a shallow warm one makes hemorrhoids more tolerable, so experiment and make your own decision. One mom told me she got the most relief for her hemorrhoids in the shower. She simply set the water on warm, turned her back on the nozzle, opened her cheeks, and let the water flow for a few minutes. You can also cut down on the pain by simply tucking the hemorrhoids back into the rectum, if possible.

Like they do with an episiotomy, Tucks and witch hazel–soaked pads will soothe itching and soreness. A hemorrhoid ointment like Preparation H (made with a variety of interesting ingredients, such as shark liver oil) will also relieve pain and itching, lubricate the area, and, as the commercials always say, "help shrink hemorrhoidal tissues." Many women make their first-ever purchase of Preparation H in the weeks after childbirth. (Incidentally, I read an article not long ago disproving the popular urban myth that Preparation H is the most shoplifted item in the United

States because people are too embarrassed to buy it.) Gynecologist Neysa Whiteman thinks a hemorrhoid ointment containing cortisone—such as Anusol HC—works even better than those without it; this type of medication has recently become available without a prescription.

Hard stools and straining aggravate hemorrhoids, so it's important to ward off constipation (see the following section for tips on how to do this).

If you're still really bothered by hemorrhoids several weeks after childbirth, you may want to look into a permanent solution. Some doctors use cryosurgery, freezing a hemorrhoid with liquid nitrogen, which eventually causes it to drop off; others inject a chemical that shrinks the enlarged vein. A more popular method that also makes the hemorrhoid eventually fall off involves the doctor tightly fastening a tiny rubber band around the hemorrhoid. (This is not as painful as it sounds, one satisfied mom told me.) All of the above procedures are usually performed in the doctor's office.

A hemorrhoidectomy is the surgical removal of a hemorrhoid and requires a hospital stay. Some doctors have also begun removing hemorrhoids with a laser; this is an outpatient procedure.

Constipation. The primary ways to ease or prevent constipation are to get up and get moving as soon as you can after childbirth in order to put your system into "drive," to drink six to eight glasses of water a day to keep bowel movements soft, and to eat a high-fiber diet because high-fiber foods move more easily through the large intestine. In the bread and cereals category, high-fiber choices include bran cereals and muffins and whole-grain or whole wheat baked goods. High-fiber veggies include spinach, celery, cabbage, lettuce, carrots, and turnips. Apples, plums, apricots, figs, and prunes are among the highest-fiber fruits. My own personal favorite food, popcorn, is also relatively high in fiber.

If you still have constipation problems despite these measures, try an enema or a laxative (but get your doctor's okay first for the laxative if you're breastfeeding and for the enema if you had a major tear or what's called a fourth-degree episiotomy).

Varicose veins and spider veins. Varicose veins tend to improve after childbirth, but they don't go away completely. If yours cause problems for you—itchiness, soreness, or a feeling of fatigue in the legs are common complaints—you may want to try wearing support hose or the even heavier-duty elastic stockings (also called compression stockings), which you may be able to purchase at your hospital pharmacy (or try a surgical supply store). It also helps to spend a few minutes every day sitting with your legs up so that they are higher than your heart. This helps empty the blood from the legs. Exercises that work the legs are also helpful because they pump blood from the legs to the heart. If you've had a stationary bicycle gathering cobwebs in the garage for years, this is the perfect use for it.

One solution to both varicose and spider veins is sclerotherapy, performed by a dermatologist. In this office procedure, the veins are injected with a saline solution, which causes them to swell shut. Because blood isn't circulating through the veins, they cease to be visible. The process takes just a few minutes and costs between $75 and $125. Three or four sessions are usually necessary. A friend's mother has had sclerotherapy, and she told me it doesn't hurt; each shot feels no worse than a "little pinch." Apparently, the biggest complaint people have about this procedure is that it isn't necessarily permanent. The veins can come back a few years later.

If varicose veins are particularly large, you may need surgery that requires a hospital stay, although Luis Navarro, M.D., a senior clinical instructor of surgery at the Mount Sinai School of Medicine in New York City, told *Parents* magazine that surgery is necessary in less than one-quarter of all varicose vein cases. The surgery, which provides a permanent cure, usually involves removing (or "stripping") the damaged vein or tying it off (also known as ligation) and leaves small scars on the legs. Often, surgery and sclerotherapy are combined.

Breast engorgement. If you aren't planning to breastfeed, you can relieve the pain of engorgement with ice packs and over-the-counter pain medications. It also helps to wear a very snug bra; a stretchy, flattening exercise bra that doesn't allow much bounce is a good choice. Don't squeeze out any milk or otherwise stimulate your nipples, because this just keeps the milk production process in gear. Whiteman says a prescription drug called bromocryptine can be helpful in drying up the milk.

If you are planning to breastfeed, use *heat* instead of cold to relieve the engorgement by getting the milk flowing out of the breasts. Just standing in the shower and letting hot water run down your chest helps a lot, or use a heating pad or a washcloth dunked in hot water. Some women find relief by massaging the breasts from the top toward the nipple; this promotes the letdown reflex that's key to getting the milk out of the breasts. You may need to hand-express milk from the breast to relieve engorgement; an inexpensive (ten dollars to fifteen dollars) manual breast pump can get you started.

Once you've established breastfeeding, nurse frequently to prevent engorgement. (Don't worry, your baby will want to nurse a lot more frequently than the once every four hours the hospital leads you to believe he will!) Alternate the breast you start with at each feeding, since the baby will take the most milk from that one, and keep track of which breast went first. My friend Janice found a great way to do this: She simply moved a cheap ring (her fingers were still too swollen to allow wearing her wedding ring) from hand to hand. An alternative is to move a safety pin from one bra strap to the other.

Sore nipples. One common cause of sore nipples is that the baby isn't latching on properly. Make sure she is sucking the *entire* nipple (which includes the areola, the dark area around the nipple tip) and that her bottom lip isn't also being pulled into her mouth as she nurses. When the baby is finished, put your finger into the corner of her mouth to break the suction before she pulls away.

Don't wash your breasts with soap—use only water—and try to keep the nipples dry. Nursing pads or even pieces of cut-up cloth diaper worn inside your bra will absorb moisture (and prevent that "leaky look" on your clothes). Irritated and cracked nipples are really helped by exposure to air. If you can't walk around the house wearing just a nursing bra with the flaps down, then at least try to spend a few hours a day with the flaps down under a big, baggy shirt.

Commercial breast creams can be soothing. Your doctor will probably recommend something that doesn't have to be washed off and that won't hurt the baby. A small amount of Vitamin E oil is a popular remedy, as is lanolin, but you can't use lanolin if you're allergic to wool since that's what it's made from.

In cases of really severe soreness or cracking, when a mother is about to give up on breastfeeding altogether because of the pain, a doctor will often recommend the use of a nipple shield or will advise pumping into a bottle for twenty-four to forty-eight hours. In either case, there is no direct contact with the nipple, so it has time to heal. By all means, buy a breast pump or ask your doctor for a "Mr. Nipple" (as we called mine) before you throw in the towel.

If you're pregnant, you may want to toughen up your nipples in the final weeks of your pregnancy to prepare them for breastfeeding. One way to do this is to rub them gently with a towel for a minute or two after you bathe or shower; also, pull out and roll your nipples between your thumb and pointing finger for a couple of minutes in the morning and then again before you go to bed. Your obstetrician or midwife may have other suggestions.

Lower back pain. Here are ways to take the strain off your back when you do three very common new-mother activities:

• When you sit down to feed your baby, prop your feet up so that your knees are higher than your hips.

• Whenever you need to stand in one place for a while, such as to wash bottles, put one foot on a stool or, if you're standing at the sink, simply open the cupboard beneath the sink and put one foot on the ledge inside. Shift your weight on and off the raised foot and alternate the feet.

• Here's how Jan K. Richardson, director of the school of physical therapy at Slippery Rock University in Pennsylvania, says to lift a baby out of a crib (according to *Good Housekeeping*): lower one side of the crib and then lean into it while resting one knee against the side of the crib; pull the baby close to your body before standing up.

If, despite these measures, you still end up with a back-ache, try the good old "pelvic rock" exercise, which you probably learned in Lamaze class. I found this to be the best backache-relieving exercise both during and after pregnancy, and it has the added benefit of strengthening your abdominal muscles, which will in turn provide better support for your back in the future.

To do the pelvic rock, kneel on all fours, holding yourself up with elbows straight and legs slightly apart. Inhale and use your abdominal muscles to arch up your back. Tuck your head and buttocks under. As you exhale, relax your back slowly. Repeat twelve times.

Fatigue. Fatigue is not just a problem in the first few months, it's a problem of the first few *years*. One of the biggest contributors to fatigue is the lack of sleep inherent in early parenthood, so I've devoted a whole chapter to dealing with that (Chapter 4). Please read it, because getting enough uninterrupted sleep is more than half the battle. Here, however, are some non-sleep-related tips for the first several postpartum weeks. The demands of the newborn combined with the demands of your changing body will make these weeks the most fatiguing you'll ever know (unless you have a second baby).

• Act like an invalid in the first week. While our mothers stayed in the hospital for a week or two, most of today's new mothers are allotted only a *day* or two. In most cases, that's nowhere near enough time to recover from the rigors of childbirth. While you don't need to stay in bed that first week, you really do need to take it much easier than usual. One way to get this message across to the hordes who want to see the baby or to the neighbor who asks you to watch her kids "just for an hour since you're home anyway" is to *wear your bathrobe all day every day.*

You may find that your husband, in particular, needs to be educated that you are *not* yourself yet and that you are *not* yet ready to resume your former level of activity, even though you may look back to normal. Men, you see, have no physiological experience in their lives that compares to childbirth. "I heard one try to liken his experience with a kidney stone to birthing a child, but take it from a woman who's had one of each—that's utter and complete codswallop," said my friend Glenda. "There is no comparison." Comedian Robin Williams once put it this way: "As the father, you think you're sharing in the birth experience. But unless you're passing a bowling ball, I don't think so. Unless you're circumcising yourself with a chain saw, I don't think so."

One woman told me her husband came to understand and sympathize with her postpartum physical condition in one instant: "He accidentally walked in on me when I was changing my sanitary pad, and when he saw the amount of blood I was losing, his face went absolutely ghost white. I think men understand the connection between blood loss and weakness very well."

• Do accept help, but you call the shots. If your mother, mother-in-law, or some other relative or friend offers to come stay with you and help for a week or two, by all means go for it—as long as both you and your husband truly like the person. If you don't, you'll just be adding extra tension to an already stressful period of your life.

It also helps if you're clear about what this helper's role will be. Consider one mother's lament: "All my mother wanted to do was take care of the baby, but that's what *I* wanted to do," she said. "I wanted Mom to handle the household stuff. It got to the point where, whenever the baby cried, we were literally racing each other to see who could get to him first. Meanwhile, the dishes piled up until

I did them. I was constantly seething with resentment, and I think that just made the first couple of weeks harder than they would have been had my mother not come at all."

Don't leave your helper to her own devices. Besides racing you to the baby, she may end up rearranging your cupboards. Be specific about what she can do for you: "Mom, will you run a load of laundry?" or "Aunt Lillian, will you please drop off Bill's suit at the cleaners and then stop and get some milk?" And don't feel guilty about doing this. She's supposed to be there to *help*, remember?

Try not to be judgmental if you delegate a task and the "helper" (who may be your husband) does that chore differently than you do. Don't decide "it's easier for me to just do it myself." Unless something your helper is doing is wrecking your furniture, ruining your clothes, or endangering your physical health, it is almost never easier to do it yourself in those first weeks after childbirth. One mother told me that when she finally delegated the grocery shopping to her husband, "It bothered me that he'd always come home with strange, exotic, inedible cheeses and the megasizes of everything. Two years later, we still have the box of graham crackers he bought a month after our son was born. But I'd just bite my lip and tell myself 'I can live with this.' And it turned out I could."

If you're pregnant now, be aware that the chores you will probably feel least like tackling postpartum are (according to my informal poll) cooking dinner and cleaning the house. So, if you have no friend or relative to help you in that first week or two, at the very least hire a maid service to come in and clean once a week (if people ask you for suggestions, a gift certificate for such a service makes an excellent baby shower or new-baby gift) and have your husband bring home takeout or frozen dinners every single night.

• Don't be so hard on yourself. I have heard a lot of new mothers beat up on themselves. "I look like a mess, my house is a mess, and the baby screams with colic every evening from five to nine solid no matter what I do," one frazzled mother told me, for example, over the phone at six weeks postpartum.

There is no reason to feel inadequate. Look at it this way: Taking care of a baby is a full-time job; running a home is *another* full-time job. And let's face it, even in the liberated 1990s it's still wives and not husbands who are managing the home in probably 95 percent of U.S. families. Doing two full-time jobs really well is close to impossible, especially when you're not yet physically up to snuff. To remain a sane woman, you're going to have to let one of those full-time jobs slide a little, and of course you'll probably decide to let the house-related stuff do the sliding. Here's some consolation: no one who's actually been a parent expects you to have a perfect house. In fact, there's a negative connotation to too much tidiness in a house where children live. (Come on, admit it. Haven't you ever thought or gossiped about someone else, "She cares more about her furniture than her kids"?)

I'm not going to turn into Heloise on you, but I can offer one tip that, in the first two years of my daughter's life, allowed me to feel as if I was still maintaining some semblance of my prebaby household order and control. I simply placed a large, acceptably attractive receptacle (a wicker basket, copper pot, or old camptrunk) in every major room, and once a day (usually in the evening or shortly before a guest was scheduled to arrive) I'd walk through the house and toss all the clutter into these receptacles. I wouldn't bother with that stuff again until I had the energy or until I was looking for something that wasn't in its usual place.

I also think it's important to reward yourself every day in the first several weeks after childbirth. Reward yourself for simply managing to get through another day. If you find yourself dragging at noon, just anticipating the reward— say, a nap when the baby naps—can keep you going. One mom I know rewarded herself with a half-hour soak each evening in a tubful of hideously expensive bath oil. Several women I talked to, particularly those who breastfed and didn't have to worry much about calories, chose a food reward. For me, it was a nightly scoop of pralines and cream ice cream. (You still have a couple of years before you have to start setting a good example and practicing the popular parenting maxim "Never use food as a reward"!) One brand-new mother I know rewards herself with the vicarious thrill of watching "Geraldo" every afternoon. "In another year, 'Geraldo' will be completely off-limits in this household," she said, "but for now the baby is completely oblivious to the transvestites parading around and the women who shot their husbands for sleeping with their sisters."

• Make sure you're getting enough iron. If you always seem to be dragging, pregnancy and childbirth may have depleted your iron stores. Good food sources for this mineral are chicken, broccoli, and spinach, or ask your doctor if you should continue to take the iron supplement you probably took during pregnancy. Gynecologist Whiteman suggests that nursing mothers also continue to take their prenatal vitamins.

Help for the Long Run

In this section, you'll find aid for the problems you may still be suffering after the six-week "official" postpartum period has ended. Let's also look at some ways to permanently improve your new body.

Tighten Up: K Power!

Every Lamaze instructor sings the praises of Kegel exercises for pregnant women because they keep the pelvic muscles toned, and those muscles in turn provide support for the pelvic organs that are under so much strain. But many new mothers are unaware of how helpful Kegels can be *after* the baby is born. They can help an episiotomy heal, tighten a loose vagina, protect against prolapse of the uterus (the uterus sinking into the vagina), and prevent or even cure many cases of urinary incontinence (the inability to hold urine), according to La Jolla, California, obstetrician and gynecologist (OB/GYN) Stephen DiMarzo. Some doctors ask their patients to begin doing Kegels—say, twenty-five to fifty a day—within a day of childbirth. No one suggested postpartum Kegels to you? No problem. You'll see improvements even if you don't begin until several weeks or even months postpartum.

Kegels (named for their inventor, a gynecologist named Arnold Kegel) are squeezes of the perineal muscles. You can learn which muscles to squeeze by stopping your urine flow midstream.

What's wonderful about Kegels is that no one can tell that you're doing them. You can even hold a conversation while you squeeze and release. This is why DiMarzo has no qualms about asking his postpartum patients to do three hundred to four hundred Kegels a day for the first couple of postpartum months, and then to taper off, but to continue the practice of five "reps" daily throughout life.

One way to get into the habit: do your Kegels during the same activities every day. DiMarzo said, for example, that most women should be able to do one hundred to two hundred Kegels just while driving to work. (Let's see. If you hold each Kegel for one second, then release for one second, you can do thirty per minute. Imagine how smug you'll feel as you drive on the freeway secretly doing 3,600 kph while in a 55-mph zone!)

The first time I ever heard of Kegels was in high school; I was secretly reading a bestselling book written by a famous sex queen. To tighten herself up, she used to do Kegels by trying to hold a pencil in her vagina! Well, apparently because some women have trouble learning to do Kegels effectively, a company has designed a "vaginal weight" that works better than a pencil. Inserted inside the vagina like a tampon, the weighted cone gives you the feeling that you're going to lose it, which makes the pelvic floor muscles contract. That's a Kegel. These weights are quite effective; one study found that half the women who used them while awaiting urinary incontinence surgery were cured and no longer needed the surgery. (And *Ms.* magazine reports a side benefit: stronger orgasms.) You can obtain vaginal weights through your gynecologist or call the manufacturer, Dacomed, directly at (800) 235-1959.

When You Can't Hold It

I know three women (each the mother of three) who jog together every morning wearing sanitary pads because urine leaks out whenever they exercise. If after childbirth you, too, have a problem with stress incontinence (the inability to hold urine at times), you're in good company. More than 25 percent of women between the ages of thirty and fifty-nine have incontinent episodes. One-fourth of all sanitary products are purchased, in fact, because of urine flow, not menstrual flow.

Here's an even more comforting statistic: almost 80 percent of people who have this often embarrassing problem can be cured, or their condition at least significantly improved. This is why seeking treatment is important if your incontinence is upsetting you.

Usually, the first thing a doctor will suggest to remedy the problem is Kegel exercises. (See the section above for complete information.) Some other tips for minimizing the problem:

• Go to the bathroom on a regular basis, as often as every hour.

• Don't hold it. Go to the bathroom when the urge first hits you.

• Make sure the bladder is completely empty before you get up from the toilet.

Incontinence expert Katherine Jeter, Ed.D., of the self-help group called Help for Incontinent People (HIP), told *Prevention* magazine that some people have reported being more prone to incontinent episodes after they eat or drink certain things. Commonly named examples: coffee, tea, alcoholic beverages, soft drinks, milk, citrus juices and citrus fruits, sugar, corn syrup, honey, chocolate, tomatoes and tomato-based products, and highly spiced foods. She also said some HIP members have reported incontinence problems after wearing nylon underpants or even pantyhose and after using colored toilet paper, scented sanitary pads and tampons, bubble baths, perfumed douches, and/or highly alkaline or antibacterial soaps. Jeter didn't suggest avoiding all of the above, but she did suggest removing one food, beverage, or substance at a time from your life for one week in order to determine if it does, in fact, exacerbate your problem.

There are drugs that can help tighten the urinary sphincter muscle and others that suppress uninhibited bladder contractions, and you may want to ask your doctor about these. Just keep in mind that such drugs aren't permanent cures for incontinence; when you stop taking them, the incontinence may return.

If none of the above works for you, surgery can cure the problem by tightening up the pelvic-floor muscles. You shouldn't even consider such surgery till after you've completed your family, however, because the trauma of a subsequent birth can make the problem recur. Your doctor may suggest, as an alternative to surgery, a specially designed pelvic support device called a *pessary*, which is worn inside the vagina during the day. In the near future, doctors may also begin treating incontinence with a collagen injection; researchers say such an injection firms up slackened urinary tract muscles.

You can contact HIP at P.O. Box 544, Union, SC 29379, (803) 579-7900.

PMS Busters

You may remember reading in Chapter 2 that while menstrual cramps often decrease in intensity or even cease completely after pregnancy, premenstrual syndrome (PMS) usually gets worse. What a trade-off, huh?

Since nobody has proven beyond a shadow of a doubt what causes PMS, treatment of the disorder has had to focus not on curing the problem at its root but on controlling its symptoms. Incredibly, there are some 140 different symptoms, and none of us seems to have the same mix of these. If your symptoms aren't too severe, I suggest you just experiment with some of the mostly dietary changes suggested below. If PMS is really turning you into a different person for a few days a month or is otherwise severely impacting your life, you probably need medication and should see a doctor, specifically a doctor who lists PMS as one of her specialties. Where to find such doctors? They often advertise in local and regional women's publications. Also, many hospitals offer PMS seminars as a part of their community outreach programs, and the leaders of these are usually gynecologists or endocrinologists who specialize in this disorder. Ask local hospitals to send you lists of their upcoming courses. Some hospitals also have physician referral phone lines. Be sure to mention that you don't want just any gynecologist, you want a doctor who lists PMS as a specialty.

The first-line treatment for PMS usually is changes in the diet. Oregon State University studies have linked both a high-sugar diet and caffeine to PMS, so you might want to try cutting down on that sort of thing, especially during the second half of your cycle. In the sugar study, researchers found that women who drank three to five cups of fruit juice daily, for example, were more likely to have severe PMS symptoms than women who didn't have such a high sugar intake. And women who drank four to twelve beers a week (alcohol is high in sugar) were three times likelier to experience PMS than women who drank no alcohol. Annette McKay Rossignol, chairperson of the Department of Public Health at Oregon State and the leader of the study, told the *Los Angeles Times* that her team isn't sure why sugar has this effect on PMS, though she speculated that women who eat a lot of sugar may not take in adequate amounts of other foods.

In the caffeine study, the Oregon researchers found that drinking even one caffeinated beverage per day raised the rate of PMS symptoms 30 percent, and women in the study who drank seven to ten cups of cola or coffee a day were seven times more likely to have PMS symptoms.

Another dietary change that doctors often recommend is limiting salt intake. This helps to reduce fluid retention and bloating. At the height of your PMS, you may also want to avoid cabbage, cauliflower, brussels sprouts, beans, soy food, chickpeas, and raisins. All of these promote bloating because they release gas during digestion. Diet sodas are also bloaters. Other foods on the "no" list in the week or two before your period: red meat and smoked and canned foods that contain preservatives. The amino acids in the meat and chemicals in the canned stuff are thought to intensify the hormonal changes of PMS, which in turn intensify PMS mood swings.

An important U.S. Department of Agriculture study released in 1991 showed that one thing you *should* eat if you're a PMS sufferer is food rich in calcium, such as broccoli and yogurt. Women in the study who increased their daily calcium intake from 600 milligrams (the average daily consumption for most of us) to 1,300 milligrams reported significantly fewer problems with PMS symptoms such as mood swings, irritability, and depression. (As an added benefit, they also had fewer backaches, headaches, and cramps during menstruation itself—probably because calcium makes muscles less tight.) Calcium is believed to help regulate the hormones; hormonal fluctuations are thought by many experts to be responsible for PMS in the first place.

Researchers have found that another mineral with hormone-regulating power is zinc. A recent Baylor College of Medicine study found that zinc levels are significantly lower in women who have PMS than in those who don't. The researchers did caution women, however, not to go overboard on zinc supplements, because this mineral can be very toxic. A better idea is to eat zinc-rich foods such as poultry and fish.

While we're on the topic of supplements, some doctors suggest that their PMS patients take extra Vitamin B-6 during the premenstrual phase of their cycles. Though no scientific studies have proved it, extra B-6 supposedly decreases PMS depression. Use caution here, too, however: never take more than three hundred milligrams of this vitamin per day because high doses over long periods can cause neurological problems. Another supplement some PMS sufferers swear by is Oil of Evening Primrose, which is available at health food stores. To find out how best to use these supplements, you may wish to consult a naturopath (a specialist in treating problems with naturally occurring elements rather than with drugs) or an M.D. with a reputation for a holistic approach to health care.

One other recommendation on the diet front: eat a complex-carbohydrate–rich snack or meal every three hours while you have PMS. Complex carbs—or "starchy" foods, as people used to call them—are anything made with whole-grain flour, oats, rice, barley, quinoa, or potatoes. Small, carbohydrate-rich meals make for a stable blood-sugar level, and a stable blood-sugar level makes for the most efficient usage of progesterone. Many prominent PMS researchers believe that a shortage of that particular hormone in the days before menstruation causes PMS.

For that reason, one treatment for severe PMS is progesterone suppositories (progesterone taken orally, according to British physician and PMS expert Katharina Dalton, is not effective against PMS). In her book *Once a Month*, Dalton talked about how once a woman with PMS starts using progesterone, "it is often difficult to recognize her as the same person."

San Diego gynecologist Neysa Whiteman agreed. "In

the U.S., progesterone as a treatment for PMS has never been proven effective, and many experts feel it's no better than a placebo. But years ago, I must have had hundreds of patients using progesterone, and they swore up and down that it was the best thing they'd ever done," Whiteman said. "It changed their lives, and it made them feel wonderful. And how can you argue with that?"

She also said that after six months or a year, most of these women would go off the progesterone, classifying themselves cured. "I don't know whether the regimen permanently changed their hormonal balance, whether it helped them deal with the PMS problems more effectively, or what," Whiteman said. "But they stopped needing it."

Curiously, far fewer women with PMS in the 1990s ask Whiteman about progesterone therapy, or seem interested when she brings it up, than did PMS sufferers in the 1980s. She speculates that may be because women coming into their own worst PMS years don't know about progesterone therapy, and that may be because magazines and newspapers have sort of abandoned PMS as a topic and turned their focus to menopause instead.

Not that progesterone is twenty-four–carat gold. Some scientists have expressed concern that it may elevate a woman's cancer risks. And it can have some unpleasant side effects—acne for example. It can even cause depression on its own.

Whiteman said that some gynecologists and endocrinologists these days are recommending that their PMS patients take "monophasic" birth control pills, which provide a low but steady dose of both progesterone and estrogen. The theory here is that while you're on this pill your hormone levels are consistent instead of fluctuating, the situation many blame for PMS.

Now let's switch from the reproductive hormone theorists to the brain hormone theorists. Scientists at Baylo. College of Medicine in Houston discovered in a study that 70 percent of women with PMS experience a rise in the level of endorphins at midcycle, followed by a plunge in those levels before their periods. Endorphins are brain hormones that are natural painkillers and mood boosters, so the researchers speculated that if they could keep endorphin levels constant, they could prevent PMS. To do this, they gave twenty women with PMS the drug Trexan, which blocks endorphin from binding with its receptors. Fourteen of these women experienced great relief of both physical and psychological symptoms. Research on this drug continues; we may even see it on the market before we hit menopause and don't need it. Incidentally, one natural way to keep those endorphin levels high, say Whiteman and other PMS specialists, is with regular exercise. Endorphins are the source of that euphoric state long-distance runners call the "runner's high."

Researchers at the University of California at San Diego are also working on a link between brain hormones and PMS. They've discovered that women who suffer from premenstrual depression secrete lower amounts of a brain hormone called melatonin, which is commonly released at night. Motivated by a desire to develop treatments that don't involve taking medicine, the UCSD scientists found that exposing women to extra bright light during the premenstrual phase relieved their PMS-related depression, sometimes for months.

Kathryn Lee, a nurse and researcher at the University of California at San Francisco, believes PMS may be related to poor-quality sleep. "What interested me," she told *Cosmopolitan* magazine, "is that the classic PMS symptoms— fatigue, irritability, mood swings—are the same as those of sleep deprivation." Her original theory was that women with PMS were losing stages three and four sleep, the deepest sleep, in the premenstrual part of their cycle. But after watching both PMS sufferers and a control group in a sleep lab, Lee got a surprise: the PMS women slept a lot less deeply than a control group throughout the entire month, not just in the week or so before their periods. "So whatever is going on in the neurological pathway that manifests as PMS is also affecting their sleep patterns on a regular basis," she said in *Cosmo.* More research into the sleep-PMS connection is needed, but meanwhile Lee pointed out that some typical PMS treatments, such as more exercise and less caffeine, are also prescribed to combat poor sleep. (You'll find more information on improving the quality of your sleep in Chapter 4.)

Finally, in a PMS "cure" category of its own is . . . orgasm! Researchers believe orgasm can at least help to relieve PMS bloating and cramps. "Muscle contractions during orgasm force blood to flow rapidly away from the pelvic region and back into general circulation, loosening tightness," said Alfred Franger, M.D., associate professor of obstetrics, gynecology, and psychiatry at the Medical College of Wisconsin in Milwaukee, in *Redbook.*

Your PMS specialist will probably know the current status of the new treatments I described, as well as any other theories and regimens that may have been suggested since I wrote these words. Because of the recent push to devote more research to women's health concerns, PMS is a popular field of study for researchers. Perhaps we'll know the definitive cause of the disorder, and its cure, by the turn of the century.

A New and Improved Body

So you want to lose some of that "baby fat," huh? Well, the next several pages are devoted to weight loss. But don't go looking for one of those here's-what-to-eat-Monday-Tuesday-Wednesday-breakfast-lunch-dinner-one-scoop-of-cottage-cheese-six-raisins-four-ounces-chicken-no-skin diets. I'm proposing something much simpler—and much more satisfying.

Losing "Baby Fat"

In 1991, there was a revolution in the weight loss world, or, as one reporter put it, "It was a bombshell in the war on blubber." A Cornell University study concluded that people can eat all they want and still lose weight as long as the food is low in fat. The eleven-week study divided thirteen women into two groups—a group that ate as much as they wanted of low-fat foods (20 to 25 percent of their daily calories came from fat) and a group that ate a diet in which 35 to 40 percent of daily calories came from fat (the approximate amount in the average American's diet). The first group lost an average of one-half pound per week. A newspaper reporter, impressed with these results, decided to try it herself and did even better; by simply cutting as much fat as possible from her diet, she lost an average of 1¾ pounds a week. (She later did a computer analysis and found that her diet averaged 15 to 16 percent of calories from fat and 1,246 to 1,752 calories a day.)

These experiences jibe with my own. In January 1993, my husband and I decided to limit our intake of fat because his first-ever blood cholesterol test came back precipitously high. I did not radically alter our diet, but I made numerous small changes. We began to use fat-free salad dressing, for example, and to substitute plain yogurt for sour cream on baked potatoes. By the end of April, I'd lost seven pounds.

The truly wonderful thing about a low-fat, all-you-can-eat diet is that the weight loss is actually just a *bonus*. You see, this is the kind of eating style experts have for the last few years been urging all Americans to adopt because it significantly reduces your risks of getting heart disease, cancer, and a host of other ills.

Another plus: you never get that hungry, deprived feeling you get on "diets," because you get to eat all you want as long as the foods are low in fat. Bread, for example (a no-no on most traditional diets), is both filling and low-fat (as long as you leave off the butter or margarine).

It surprised many researchers that people on low-fat diets don't suffer from hunger pangs, because the conventional wisdom was that it's the fat in food that makes people feel full and satisfied. Most diet experts believed that if you eat less fat, you'll compensate by eating more of other foods. But one of the biggest bombshells of the Cornell study was that people do *not* judge fullness by fat content. They judge it by the bulk of the food consumed.

The scientific explanation for why people who limit their fat intake lose weight is that the body stores, instead of using, calories that come from fat more readily than calories from protein or carbohydrate. David Levitsky, professor of nutrition and psychology at Cornell and the chief investigator for the study, told the newspaper reporter that, basically, fat is what makes you fat. To shed the fat on your body, he said, you must reduce the amount of fat you put in your mouth. And you don't have to reduce it by much. Margaret Zurack, who's the director of nutrition at the popular Canyon Ranch spa in the Berkshires, once said that if you cut just one tablespoon of fat out of your diet every day, you'll lose ten pounds in a year.

In addition to all of the above reasons, I think a low-fat, all-you-can-eat way of life (I hate to use the word *diet* because it implies short term, and the way of eating I'm suggesting is something worth adopting for life) is perfect for mothers of young children because:

• There isn't a lot of time-consuming weighing and measuring necessary, as there is in many traditional diets.

• No food is off-limits. You don't have to beat up on yourself mentally if you succumb to a piece of chocolate cake. Just compensate by having less fat than usual for dinner—a smaller piece of meat, for example.

• The whole family can, and should, be on the same low-fat diet, so you don't have to prepare different foods for yourself. Three caveats here, however. First, if you're breastfeeding, ask your doctor if it's okay to limit fat. Some doctors don't like lactating women to lose more than one pound a week; others oppose weight loss in breastfeeders *period*. Second, ask your pediatrician if a low-fat diet is okay for your child. Many pediatricians feel fat should not be limited in the first two years of life. You may need to serve your child whole instead of nonfat milk, for example. Finally, if you have high blood pressure, you'll probably want to choose foods that are not only low in fat but low in salt, as well.

It's simple. If you opt for a low-fat, all-you-can-eat diet, you really have to keep only one number in mind: limit your fat intake to forty grams per day or less (decrease that goal number a bit if you're on the short side). This will ensure that you lose weight slowly but surely. I've included several charts (see Appendix B) with data compiled by the U.S. Department of Agriculture Human Nutrition Information Service that state the number of grams of fat (and other stuff that's not so great) in various kinds of food. You can also get fat information by reading the labels on food, but be sure you know exactly how much of the product the manufacturer is referring to. Often, to make a food appear to be less fattening, a sneaky manufacturer will base the ingredient breakdown on a serving size that would be too small for a two-year-old!

I also urge you to invest in some good low-fat cookbooks. Two that I use often are the *Sunset Low-Fat Cookbook* (Sunset Publishing Corp., Menlo Park, California) and *The Ultimate Recipe for Fitness,* by Sheila Cluff and Eleanor Brown (Fitness Publications, Ojai, California). There are also two good USDA Human Nutrition Information Service booklets that include low-fat recipes. "Preparing Foods & Planning Menus" ($2.50; item #172-V) and "Shopping for Food & Making Meals in Minutes" ($3; item #174-V) can be ordered from the Consumer Information Center, Dept. 70, Pueblo, Colorado 81009 (make checks payable to the Superintendent of Documents).

Tricks and Treats

I've gathered some favorite cooking tips from converts to the low-fat way of life:

• Salsa! Put it on the table in place of higher-fat condiments such as mayonnaise and sour cream. It's great on baked potatoes and as a "cover" for fish or chicken instead of rich sauces. And it's not only low in fat: the tomatoes and other veggies make it high in vitamins.

• Use applesauce (or other pureed fruit) instead of oil when you bake. Pumpkin and creamed corn are other fat alternatives. Use twice the amount of fruit or vegetable; if the recipe calls for ¼ cup of oil, for example, use ½ cup of applesauce. If you absolutely cannot bring yourself to cut all the fat from a baking recipe, try cutting the amount in half. Most baked goods can tolerate this reduction with little change in taste.

• Sauté vegetables in chicken broth rather than butter or margarine, each of which has a whopping eleven grams of fat per tablespoon. Water or fruit juice can also substitute for oil when you want to sauté.

• Take the skin off chicken. On a half-breast of roasted chicken, removing the skin reduces fat from eight grams to three.

• Use only the whites of eggs in recipes. (Two egg whites equal one whole egg.) You save five grams of fat per egg yolk. Alternative: try a fat-free egg substitute.

• Cut the fat off meat. When you trim the fat off a three-ounce piece of broiled sirloin steak, you're also trimming the fat you consume from fifteen grams to six.

• When you toss pasta, a fairly decent substitute for oil is simply a few tablespoons of the water you cooked it in. If you *must* have oil, put it in a water bottle and spray it on the pasta. You'll use less. Same goes for sautéing with oil: you'll save if you spray the pan rather than pour the oil in.

• Choose pourable salad dressings rather than the jar type, or thin the jar variety with sherry, raspberry, rice-wine, or balsamic vinegar. Substitute low-fat yogurt or whipped cottage cheese for the sour cream in homemade salad dressings (this also works with dips) and replace mayonnaise with the low-fat or fat-free variety. Try the fat-free varieties of salad dressings. (I've found the fat-free "ranch"-type dressings to be particularly good.)

You really do need to be especially careful about salad dressings. A recent USDA Human Nutrition Information Service study found that *salad dressing is the number one source of fat in the diet of American women between the ages of nineteen and fifty.* According to researchers, most regular salad dressings add 5.2 grams of fat, about 47 calories, a day to a woman's diet. Over the course of a year, that adds up to more than 17,000 calories, or five pounds of fat.

• Try the fat-free varieties of other foods, too. You will be amazed at the fat-free foods that are now available—even potato chips! Some of these "imposters" are disappointing, but most are reasonable facsimiles, and a few are downright delicious and virtually indistinguishable from their fatted counterparts. Some of the fat-free, refrigerated, ready-to-eat puddings are examples of the latter. Steve and I are also addicted to Entenmann's Fat Free Chocolate Brownie Cookies, which include chunks that feel and taste exactly like chocolate chips but can't be. (And we have thus far resisted reading the label, because we really don't want to know just what they are!)

Eating Out

When you haven't prepared the meal yourself, it can be difficult to figure out how much fat you're getting. Here's help.

Appetizers. Your best choices are raw vegetables or fruit or steamed seafood. Bread or bread sticks without butter or margarine are also fine. Avoid or limit your consumption of crackers, dips, tortilla chips, and batter-fried cheese sticks, vegetables, or chicken pieces. Perhaps the *worst* possible appetizer you can order is fried potato skins that come laden with sour cream, cheese, and bacon bits. These probably pack thirty grams of fat per serving.

Translating "menu-ese." Knowing how to translate menu terms can help you zero in on the good, low-fat items to order:

Watch out for these high-fat terms:

Butter	**Cream**	**Gravy**
buttered	creamed	in its own gravy
buttery	creamy	pan gravy
	in cream sauce	with gravy
	hollandaise	

Cheese	**Fried**	**Other**
au gratin	batter-fried	breaded
in cheese sauce	deep-fried	escalloped
	French-fried	pastry
	pan-fried	rich
		scalloped

Look for these lower-fat terms:

broiled	poached	steamed
grilled	roasted	stir-fried

On the side. At the salad bar, avoid or take only minute quantities of bacon bits, eggs, cheese, and nuts. At the table, always ask that any sour cream, cream sauces, gravies, and salad dressings be served on the side. One idea for salad dressing: just dip the tines of your fork in it, then take a bite of lettuce. Or ask if you may have lemon juice or vinegar and (a little bit of) oil instead of salad dressing.

Ethnic choices. Here are your best low-fat bets when it comes to foreign fare. Japanese: sashimi. Mexican: chicken or fish burritos, enchiladas, or fajitas; rice and beans (unless they're refried). Indian: chicken tandoori. Pizza: vegetarian (never order extra cheese). Chinese: shrimp with snow peas, moo goo gai pan, which is chicken with vegetables (or order the seafood variety of this), or beef with broccoli. Italian: stick with dishes prepared with tomato-based sauces rather than those covered with cream sauces or cheese ("parmigiana").

Fast food. Go with the smallest single-patty hamburger (or the new "extra-lean" burger some fast-food restaurants offer) and hold the cheese, bacon, and/or creamy sauces. A roast beef sandwich is even leaner than a burger, as is a broiled chicken or fish sandwich. Breaded fish and chicken sandwiches, on the other hand, are higher in fat than are plain burgers, especially when you top them with cheese, tartar sauce, or mayonnaise.

Losing Your "Fat Tooth"

You may never lose your *sweet* tooth, but according to a four-year study of more than two thousand women, you probably will lose your taste for fat after a few months of limiting your fat intake. Researchers at the Fred Hutchinson Cancer Research Center at the University of Washington found that many of the women in the study who had cut their fat intake to about 25 percent of their total daily calories reported that, within about six months of changing their eating habits, they found fatty foods unpleasant to eat. So hang in there if you find yourself missing donuts.

The Exercise Factor

You don't have to exercise to lose weight. However, keep two things in mind if you've cut down on the fat in your diet but intend to remain a couch potato: (1) you'll lose *more* weight if you also exercise and (2) while cutting fat will help you drop pounds, such a change in diet will not tighten up your tummy, whittle your waist, or harden your hips. You can be thin, even underweight, and still be flabby. That's where exercise comes in.

Videos and Other Fitness Programs

For the new mother—for *any* mother with a child under age five—the problem with exercise is finding the time and energy to do it. So I'm not going to suggest you sign up for three-times-a-week aerobics classes at your local fitness center. Such classes not only require commitments of time, energy, and money but also may induce guilt, especially if you work outside the home. One working mom I know explained her reason for not signing up at the family-oriented fitness center that is literally right around the corner from her house: "I already feel like I'm not spending enough time with my baby." If you can manage to fit in formal exercise classes, more power to you. Lots of fitness centers and hospitals offer postpartum exercise classes (there's now even a step aerobics class dubbed "Step Moms"), and many offer childcare at low or no cost. If you've never taken a formal exercise class before, my friend Janice recommends you choose a hospital-sponsored course over one held at a commercial fitness center. "I tried both, and I felt more self-conscious as an aerobics rookie at the fitness center, because most of the other new moms there had been enthusiastic aerobics junkies before they were pregnant," she said.

I'm not a great advocate of video fitness programs either. When I was pregnant, I bought a video designed for pregnant women and did it religiously for two weeks. At the end of that time, I was so bored with it I wanted to scream (which is, I'm sure, a built-in problem with any fitness video). I was certain that if I heard the music that accompanies the exercises just one more time, I would go stark raving crackers.

When Madeline was about one, I tried video again, arising at 6:30 (a half-hour earlier than usual) each morning to follow along with an aerobics instructor on a PBS television program before Madeline got up. Again my participation lasted only two weeks. I simply came to the conclusion that losing that extra half-hour of sleep in the morning was doing my psyche more harm than the aerobics were doing my body good.

I rented another fitness video for a few weeks when Madeline was two. Once again, wipeout. She would either jump on my stomach as I tried to do curl-ups or head off for some distant corner of the house—and then get alarmingly quiet. Either way, I couldn't continue.

If you are more disciplined or less easily bored than I am, I can give you a couple of recommendations on the formal exercise front. First, if you're looking for a good book, two mothers whose opinions I greatly value—Anne Fehlman, who teaches exercise classes for expectant and new mothers in southern California and is a personal fitness trainer specializing in new mothers, and Kathie Davis, the founder and executive director of the San Diego–based IDEA, International Association of Fitness Professionals—both highly recommend the book *Essential Exercises for the Child-Bearing Year*, by Elizabeth Noble; it includes both pregnancy and postpartum exercises.

Regarding fitness videos, it's difficult to make specific recommendations, since I'm certain readers of this book are at widely divergent fitness levels and have widely divergent tastes. My best advice is to send for Collage Video's

"Complete Guide to Exercise Videos" catalog. (It's free if you send your name and address to Exercise Video Catalog, Dept. G, 5390 Main St., NE, Minneapolis, MN 55421.) This guide gives detailed, objective descriptions of hundreds of exercise videos and indicates how each video was rated by twelve independent sources (including *Shape*, *Lears*, and *Good Housekeeping* magazines). You can select a video not only by the ratings source you trust most but by your level of fitness and by the style of exercise you like. In addition to a huge variety of standard aerobics and toning programs, the catalog includes workouts for step-bench, ballet, stretch, yoga, tai chi, stress relief, and stationary bicycling, and there are special sections for special circumstances. There's a section detailing pregnancy/postpartum videos, for example. How does Collage make its money? Selling by mail order the videos it lists in its guide.

Take a Walk

My own personal salvation in terms of toning has been exercises I can do while I'm doing other things (see the next section); in terms of overall fitness, it has been walking. The benefits and advantages of putting your child in a stroller and embarking on a brisk walk are just amazing. For one, it's something you can do *with* your baby—no guilt or anxiety about being away from her; no babysitter required. For another, you can do it in any weather—if it rains, just pack the stroller in your trunk and head for the nearest indoor shopping mall. You can also do it within days of childbirth; if you start slow and easy, you don't have to wait the traditional six weeks like you do for most exercise programs. "It's also very good for toning the abdomen and lower body," according to Fehlman. Also, I came across a study done at Loma Linda University showing that women who walk regularly are able to fight off colds and flu twice as fast as those who don't. And, according to the Rand Corporation in Santa Monica, California, if you're an otherwise sedentary person, every mile you walk will add twenty-one minutes to your life. Why? Because, among other things, it improves your cardiovascular fitness.

Best of all, walking is a terrific calorie burner and pound dropper. Here are the statistics I found (keep in mind they can vary slightly based on your weight, how far and fast you walk, and whether you walk in a flat or hilly area): If you walk at the rate of three miles per hour or one mile every twenty minutes (and that's considered a leisurely pace) every day, you can lose two pounds a month without changing your diet. If you combine the walks with a 300-calorie-per-day cut in food intake, you'll drop four pounds per month. If you walk faster (about four miles per hour) you'll use 400 to 500 calories per hour; and going even faster or going up hills will burn up even more.

Want a real-life example? My friend Sharon Whitley embarked upon a walking program about 4½ months ago. She walks five to seven times a week, about 2.5 miles per day through a neighborhood that is mildly hilly in sections. She finishes in forty to forty-five minutes. And she's lost ten pounds so far without altering her diet.

When you step out with the stroller, you also do your baby a favor. She'll be getting fresh air, sunshine, a change of scenery. When she gets older, you can make your walks with her educational, too. When Madeline began to talk, for example, I pointed out objects along our route and asked her to name them. When she reached preschool age, we made up more "advanced" walking activities, such as finding all the letters of the alphabet via the license plates on parked cars.

If you do decide to walk as your avenue for getting in

shape, try to do so at a pace that makes your heart pump but not thump; you should be able to hold a conversation. How long should you walk, and how often? According to IDEA, you need to exercise for twenty minutes two to three times a week to maintain fitness. To *improve* fitness, you need to increase the frequency to three to four times a week and the duration to thirty minutes. And if you are also hoping to lose excess fat gained during pregnancy, you should try for at least four or five thirty-minute sessions a week.

A variation on walking is roller-skating. If you have a rink in your community, it may offer a "stroller-skating" morning once a week during which moms (or dads) are invited to skate to music while pushing baby in a stroller. We have a rink with such a program about two miles from home, and I once overheard some moms in a local park discussing what fun they'd had. I bet they didn't know that they were also burning off eleven calories per minute.

Another way to get your walking or other exercise in is to do it in the morning while your husband gets ready to go to work *and* watches the baby. (You do two things at once all the time; he can learn, too!) A friend of mine started this program when her baby was one and has worked up to a two-mile run three times a week. Other moms do co-op sitting while exercising: two moms watch the kids while a third mom exercises for half an hour; the next half hour, mom number two takes a turn. (You can also alternate on a daily basis.)

Exercises You Can Do
While You're Doing Other Things

For tightening the abdominal muscles to flatten your stomach. I got this tummy tightener from fitness expert

Sheila Cluff: just "hold it in." "Make a habit of contracting your abdominal muscles whenever you think about it," said Cluff, who owns two southern California fitness spas (The Oaks at Ojai and The Palms at Palm Springs). "You can do this exercise any place and any time—while cooking dinner, for example." To start, she said, contract your stomach muscles for a slow count of ten, relax, and repeat, remembering to check and correct your posture at the same time and to breathe deeply.

To tone up the butt. This one comes from Cluff's book, *The Ultimate Recipe for Fitness.* Whenever you climb the stairs, pretend you're holding a gold coin between your cheeks and don't drop it till you reach the top. A friend of mine, who doesn't have stairs at home, does a lesser but still effective variation of this: Whenever she's doing the "hold it in," she also clenches her buttocks. "I do this all the time when I'm waiting in line," she said. "As long as you're wearing a fairly full dress or a long, baggy shirt, no one's the wiser!"

To trim the thighs. An exercise I found in *Good House-keeping* can be done while you're on the phone. Stand with your back against a wall and walk your feet out till your heels are about twelve inches from the wall. Keeping your back straight, slowly bend your knees and slide your back down the wall till you're in a sitting position and your thighs are just about parallel to the floor. Hold the position for thirty seconds, then repeat. Try to work up to one minute.

And if you have stairs, here's another of Sheila Cluff's funny but effective ideas: Waddle up the stairs with a wiggle like Charlie Chaplin, with your knees flexed, your pelvis tucked. This is excellent, she said, for the inner thighs.

To deal with droopy breasts. No exercise will actually make your breasts sag less, but you can make them *appear* to be a little larger and perkier by building up the pectoral muscles behind them. One way to do this is with an isometric exercise. Here's one I often do in the car while waiting at stoplights: Put your left palm on the *side* (not the front) of the steering wheel at the nine o'clock position. Put your right palm on the side of the wheel at the three o'clock position. Now press them toward each other as hard and for as long as you can.

Housework Counts!

If you come to the end of the day without having fit in any exercise, don't be too hard on yourself, especially if you did a lot of housework. According to *Glamour* magazine, when you do various household tasks vigorously, you *are* getting exercise. Window washing, food shopping, or mopping, for example, burns 3.7 calories per minute—the exercise equivalent of doing jumping jacks. Sweeping or dusting uses 3.8 calories per minute—the exercise equivalent of roller-skating. Waxing and/or scrubbing floors is good for 6.8 calories per minute—equal to low-impact aerobics. And vacuuming is a real workout: 7 calories per minute, or like walking at a pace of three miles per hour. Outdoors, raking leaves is good for 5 calories a minute.

Surgical Solutions

Only as a last resort do most women consider surgery to correct postpregnancy problems. (Please read Chapter 10 before you call a plastic surgeon!) The surgeries to correct hemorrhoids, varicose veins, and stress incontinence are described earlier in this chapter. Here are procedures that remedy other problems.

Anterior and Posterior Colporrhaphy

Colporrhaphy is the medical term for surgical vaginal repair. In this surgery, incisions are made, and the fibrous tissue layers of the vagina are tightened up with sutures. The surgery results in an overall strengthening of the vagina: it tightens the vaginal opening, elevates the bladder, and pushes down the rectum. This procedure requires anesthesia and a hospital stay of about three days and can cost anywhere from $1,500 to $3,000 (the actual price, as well as the cost of other procedures described in this section, depends on the length and complexity of the operation, the anesthesia used, and the area of the country in which the surgery is performed).

OB/GYN DiMarzo told me he discourages such surgery when a woman's only complaint is vaginal looseness (not accompanied by rectal or bladder problems), because this problem can often be improved with pelvic exercises (e.g., Kegels) alone.

Augmentation Mammaplasty

Augmentation mammaplasty is surgery to enlarge the breasts with implants. The most popular implants used to be those filled with silicone; however, because the Food and Drug Administration has concerns about the safety of silicone implants, the agency has restricted their use. Most women seeking mammaplasty today receive saline (salt water) filled implants. Incisions are made underneath the breast, around the nipple, or in the underarm area (surgeon and patient decide where), and a pocket for the implant is then created beneath either the chest muscle or the breast. There is some scarring. The surgery, which lasts about two hours under local or general anesthesia, usually requires a patient to take two or three days off work, and to refrain from exercise and heavy lifting for three to four weeks. Costs usually run between $2,000 and $3,500.

James Pietraszek, a La Jolla, California, plastic surgeon, once told me that half of his augmentation patients seek the surgery because of postpartum atrophy, the shrinking of the breast tissue after pregnancy and childbirth (read "Breasts" in Chapter 2). "Actually, these patients are very good candidates for implants because the breast skin has already been stretched out and will readily accommodate an implant and look very natural right away," he said. According to the American Society of Plastic and Reconstructive Surgeons, implants have no effect on one's ability to nurse later on, though implant leaking can be a problem, according to other experts.

Keep in mind that while saline implants apparently aren't as risky as the silicone kind, complications may still arise. So, while they are still available at this writing, they also have come under FDA review. Daniel Baker, M.D., associate professor of plastic surgery at New York University Medical Center, told *McCall's* that besides the fact that saline implants can leak, "scar tissue can cause hardening of the breast, necessitating removal." There is also concern that implants might make breast cancer detection more difficult.

You may have heard of some new procedures in which implants are made from skin, muscle, and fat from the patient's own lower back or abdomen. However, because these surgeries are far more complicated (and expensive) than simple implant surgery, carry higher surgical risks, and require much longer hospital stays and recovery periods, they are generally considered only by mastectomy patients seeking reconstruction.

Mastoplexy

Also known as a breast lift, a mastoplexy raises and recontours sagging breasts. The surgeon removes excess skin from the lower part of the breast, and the nipple, areola, and underlying tissue are moved up to a new and higher position. The patient wears a supportive bra for several weeks after surgery. The surgery (which takes about two hours) costs between $1,500 and $5,000, usually requires general anesthesia, and leaves scars where the incisions were made around and below the nipples.

Abdominoplasty

Surgery to remove excess abdominal skin and to tighten the underlying musculature is called abdominoplasty. It has a cute nickname, the "tummy tuck," but it is major abdominal surgery. One common abdominoplasty approach is to make a horizontal cut just above the pubic area. A second cut frees the belly button from the surrounding skin so it can be put aside for later use. The skin is separated from the abdominal wall and elevated above the rib cage. Loose tissue that covers the abdomen's large vertical muscle is pulled toward the center of the abdomen and sewn together. The previously elevated skin is lowered, and the surgeon removes the excess and makes a small opening for the belly button. The belly button is put in its new place, and incisions are closed with stitches. After the surgery, which costs $2,000 to $6,000 or more, the patient must stay in the hospital for two to three days with hips bent to reduce tension on the abdomen and then must avoid overactivity and straining for up to a month.

Liposuction

In liposuction, the most popular cosmetic surgery of the 1990s, concentrated deposits of fat (usually in the abdomen, hips, thighs, or under the chin) are literally vacuumed out via small tubes that are inserted into the body through small incisions. There is usually bruising and swelling (which fades in four to six weeks), and the patient is required to wear a bandage or special girdle for up to six weeks to help the skin shrink and heal smoothly and evenly. The procedure costs between $1,500 and $6,000 and usually requires general anesthesia. Most patients go home the same day but need a couple of days of rest to recover and must wait at least four weeks before doing any strenuous exercise. The best candidates for liposuction are people with fat deposits they can't get rid of in spite of exercise and weight loss.

CHAPTER FOUR

GETTING A GOOD
NIGHT'S SLEEP

"The first two years after my son was born were like a blur
to me," said Brenda, a graphic artist in Los Angeles and
the mother of Nicholas, now three. "I remember watching
the Grammy Awards with my husband one night and
being stunned by the realization that I'd never before
heard a single song that was nominated. I decided that new
motherhood was so all-consuming that I'd lost track of the
rest of the world around me."

Then Brenda and her husband took the first vacation
they'd had since before Nicholas was born. Leaving the
baby at her mother's house, they drove up the coast and
spent a week lying around a resort near Santa Barbara.

"When I got home it was like I'd put on a new pair of
glasses. Everything seemed sharper, more vibrant," Brenda
said. "I felt like my old self. And that's when I realized that
I hadn't been in a maternal daze as much as I'd been in a
fog of fatigue! I was amazed at the difference getting all of
my sleep could make."

There are two big myths out there among the uninitiated. The first is that once a baby begins to "sleep through the night" at around three months, you're home free, back to eight or nine blissful uninterrupted hours snuggled spoon fashion with your hubby. Well, dream on! What people never warn you about is that sleeping through the night for a baby usually means sleeping from midnight to 5 A.M.

And here's the other real eye-opener: thanks to teething, fevers, nightmares, and other nocturnal nuisances, it's often difficult for a mother to get enough good-quality sleep even long past the Gerber years. When my daughter Madeline was getting her second molars at age 2½, for example, there were nights when she cried out in her sleep fourteen times—about twice an hour. Though I was usually able to go back to sleep each time, I always woke up exhausted. It's like a form of torture, and there's no end in sight: In 1990, one of my sisters told me she had not slept for more than five hours a night since the first of her three children was born in 1979.

We're finally getting some scientific backing (from researchers who have toddlers at home, no doubt) that most mothers—and not just the mothers of newborns—do not get enough sleep. Michigan State University researchers found, for example, that women who work and have children under age three average almost an hour less of sleep per night than their male counterparts, who manage to fit in between seven and eight hours.

Five or six hours of sleep is not enough. Yes, Oprah Winfrey often boasts that she sleeps only four hours a night, and Martha Stewart (the party planning whiz) chooses to sleep only five. But scientists say the vast majority of us need between seven and eight hours and some need even more.

Incredibly, science still hasn't definitively answered the question of why we need to sleep in the first place. Some researchers theorize that sleep restores brain function, that it's sort of like recharging a car battery; others think sleep's purpose is to give tired body tissue time to recover. Much more is known about what happens when the body is *deprived* of sleep. Some of the effects of sleep deprivation are obvious: you feel fatigued, sleepy, and have less energy. But many other effects on your life are insidious, according to Milton Erman, M.D., head of the Sleep Disorders Center at Scripps Clinic in La Jolla, California. "It's hard for people to fully appreciate the impact sleep loss is having on them," Erman said. "But losing even just an hour or two a night can sabotage both physical and psychological performance."

One of the first things to go when you're sleep deprived is creative thinking. Your memory and ability to concentrate also aren't as good. You become clumsier at simple tasks, and your dexterity may decline to the point where a childproof cap becomes motherproof, as well. Your reaction time is slower. You are much more likely to make mistakes, and some can be dangerous. You know how the labels on medicines warn you not to operate machinery if you feel drowsy? Whenever I used to read that, I always pictured a guy running a forklift. Now I picture myself drowsily reaching into a plugged-in toaster with a fork. It's something I found myself doing recently after a four-hour night. Some investigators even believe the space shuttle disaster was the result of a decision made by a sleep-deprived person. And the Department of Transportation estimates that forty thousand traffic accidents a year may be related to sleep deprivation.

Sleep deprivation affects your mood as well as your performance. Erman said it's easy to become moody, irritable, and even depressed when you're tired. Some recent research suggests that the link between sleep loss and the blues lies in the reduced amount of REM (rapid eye movement) sleep. REM sleep is the sleep that gives us dreams, and scientists believe that the processing of emotions and memories that we do through dreaming is important to our emotional health. That's why cutting REM sleep short, a natural consequence of not getting enough sleep overall, may make you feel blue and crabby.

Renata Shafor, M.D., a neurologist and the director of the Sleep Disorders Center at Harbor View Medical Center in San Diego, said sleep-deprivation depression is sometimes so mild that people don't perceive it as depression. "You may not feel blue," Shafor said, "but you might begin to drop hobbies or to lose interest in some of the other things you used to enjoy."

Researchers at the Sleep Disorders Clinic at Toronto Western Hospital are also uncovering compelling evidence linking sleep and the immune system. The researchers suspect that if you're sleep deprived, you may be more susceptible to invading bacteria and viruses.

Sleep deprivation, by the way, is cumulative. Its ill effects increase with each subsequent night that your sleep is shortened. When we burned the proverbial candle at both ends back in the old days, before we had children, by sleeping in on weekends we could make up somewhat for the "sleep debt" incurred during the week. This extra rest was enough to tide us over into the middle of the next hectic work week before insufficient sleep once again began to take its toll. Erman said this is the main reason so many people in the work world perform better on Tuesdays than they do on Fridays.

Of course, now that you do have children you're savvy to the fact that they don't give a whit if it's Monday or

Saturday—it's all the same to their little body clocks. They want to get up *now*, and you can't exactly just swing them out of the crib and allow them free rein of the house while you trudge back to bed to catch an extra hour or two. My husband and I were laughing (rather dryly) the other day about the fact that "sleeping in" for us these days means 7:45. If I had known that back in my college days, not only would I have been incredulous that I would someday be able to laugh at such a fate, I probably would have also been horrified enough to look into surgical sterility.

How to Cope

If you're the mother of a newborn and you're still home on maternity leave, your best bet is to try to catch up on the sleep you miss at night by taking naps in the daytime while the baby sleeps. At night, your goal should be to get at least five uninterrupted hours of sleep. Probably the easiest way to do that is to go to bed early, say around nine o'clock, and get Daddy or someone else to handle the next feeding—the one before midnight—with a bottle of formula or expressed breast milk. Then you take the middle-of-the-night feeding.

This advice goes right out the window, of course, if the newborn isn't your only child, if you go back to work, or if your kids are older. Here are some strategies for dealing with sleep deprivation in those situations.

Nap whenever and wherever you can. According to University of Ottawa neurologist and sleep researcher Roger Broughton, M.D., humans are biologically wired for one nap a day, usually in the midafternoon. Studies show that napping not only will make you feel better, it will also make you better able to concentrate and to make complex decisions. With a little resourcefulness, napping may be a luxury you can afford, even if you work outside the home. One mother, an accounts payable supervisor with a fourteen-month-old, told me her staff got so used to her taking two behind-closed-doors breaks every day to pump breast milk that no one thinks twice that she's still closing her door every afternoon between 2:30 and 3. She's in there napping, not pumping; she stopped nursing when her baby was ten months old.

Bonnie, a fashion illustrator friend of mine who lives far out on Long Island, uses her purse as a pillow to nap on the train ride home from Manhattan each afternoon.

When I worked in a big office building in the early 1980s, there was a woman who napped in her car during lunch hour. My single friends and I, on our way through the parking lot to the deli, used to squish our faces against the car windows and make hideous faces at this poor woman, who was dead to the world, and joke about how many paper clips we might be able to toss into her gaping mouth. Nowadays, of course, I feel a profound sense of sisterhood with this woman, and I rather admire her complete lack of care about what other people thought.

If you do find time for a nap, keep a few guidelines in mind. You need at least twenty minutes (thirty is better) but no more than 1½ hours. Shorter than this, Erman said, has no restorative benefits, and napping any longer than ninety minutes will make it harder to fall asleep that night and/or will make your nighttime sleep lighter. Remember that, unlike nighttime sleep, daytime sleep consists mainly of deeper, nondreaming sleep. It's the kind that's harder to wake up from, the kind you wake up from with a disoriented "where am I?" feeling. So try to allow yourself an extra five or ten minutes to fully wake up.

If you can't nap, schedule your day around the "mid-afternoon blahs." Researchers say that the urge for that midafternoon nap we're biologically wired for hits about twelve hours after the middle of nighttime sleep. Example: If you sleep from 11 to 6, the drowsiness will hit at around 2 P.M. Since alertness is low, this is not the time to schedule a job interview or a major sales presentation or to attempt to put together the five thousand pieces of a "some assembly required" toy. If you're at work, use the time to return phone calls or to meet with colleagues. At home, take the kids to the playground, go for a walk with the stroller, or do something passive, such as watching "Mister Rogers' Neighborhood."

Use your television sensibly. All of us are aware of the ill effects of too much TV. And most of us would shudder at the idea of parking a preschooler in front of the set all day so that one can do one's own thing. But using the TV as a babysitter in order to bring up your sleep quota is another thing entirely. Look at it this way: acting like a witch all day because you're sleep deprived is probably worse for a child's psyche than a little TV on weekend mornings. If you've been vigilant about limiting your preschooler's viewing during the week, there's no reason to feel guilty about turning on the cartoons on Saturday morning while you doze a couple of extra hours on the couch. If, like me, you're squeamish about cartoons and commercials (frequently one and the same), lock your channel selector on PBS. (At KPBS here in San Diego, some extravagantly benevolent programmer scheduled two straight hours of "Sesame Street" early Saturday morning and three on Sundays for the first 3½ years of Madeline's life.) Or rent videos. Pick up *Lady and the Tramp* or something similar when you rent the videos you and your husband will be watching over the weekend (since you never go out any more!). Incidentally, when grandparents and others ask for gift suggestions, put videos on your list. Every family needs a good video library.

When trying to make up for lost sleep, go to bed early rather than sleep late if you have the choice. Erman said we reset our body clocks by getting up at the same time every morning. "Sleeping later than normal disrupts your body rhythms, and that leads to a feeling of sluggishness or just general unwellness during the day," he said. Going to bed an hour or so earlier than normal, on the other hand, gives you the extra rest without the side effects.

Keep in mind that an occasional night in mom and dad's bed won't turn your child into a social deviant. You've probably heard the dire warnings: letting a child into your own bed may interfere with his recognition of himself as an independent individual, may become an addiction, and may be physically overstimulating for him. But those possibilities pale when it's 3 A.M., your child is feverish, achy, and crying, and total household sleep has amounted to forty-five minutes so far. Sometimes letting your little one crawl in between the two of you is the only way anybody is going to get any sleep. As she dozes off in a horizontal position (that seems to be some sort of rule among children), remember this: experts are more relaxed about "cosleeping" than they used to be. "It's not harmful to the child," Barton Schmitt, M.D., a pediatrician at Children's Hospital of Denver, once told me flatly. "But I advise parents not to share their bed with the child because it can become a major inconvenience to the parents." If you allow it too often, Schmitt explained, he'll *never* want to sleep by himself. But the key here is, what's too often? "I don't know of any child allowed to sleep with his parents once a week who doesn't want to do it more frequently," Schmitt said. Reserve cosleeping, he said, for illness, nightmares, or thunderstorms. Other experts, notably pediatrician/author William Sears, M.D., actually *encourage* cosleeping.

Have medicine on hand to treat the conditions that keep children from sleeping. Acetaminophen (Tylenol, Panadol, Tempra) reduces fever in children. Fever is part of the body's defense against invading viruses and bacteria, and for that reason many pediatricians are in favor of letting a moderate fever (less than 103 in infants; less than 104 in older kids) run its course without intervention. But they feel sleep is just as important to the recovery process, making a dose of acetaminophen appropriate at bedtime (and every four to six hours after that through the night if your child keeps waking up as it wears off).

The same goes for cough suppressants. Most pediatricians will ask you not to try to suppress a productive (mucus-producing) cough during the day but are in favor of giving the kid a break at night.

If your child is prone to ear infections, it's a good idea to ask your pediatrician to prescribe eardrum-numbing drops that you can use until you can get to the doctor for antibiotics. One of my sisters conservatively estimates that this particular product has saved her from twenty-five sleepless nights.

There's no law that says toddlers and preschoolers must be in bed by 8 P.M. "My mother was scandalized to hear that we let our two-year-old stay up every night till ten," a mother told me, "until she invited Maura to spend the weekend at her house. She tucked Maura in at eight—and

Maura was jumping on Grandma's bed at five the next morning."

Richard Ferber, M.D., the director of the Center for Pediatric Sleep Disorders at Boston Children's Hospital, told me you can adjust children's body clocks so that they'll wake up later by putting them to bed later. But it won't work unless you make *everything* in the schedule later (lunch, afternoon nap, dinner, etc.). And you have to make the change gradually. In other words, make the entire schedule fifteen minutes later this week, another fifteen minutes later next week, and so on.

Work out equitable sleep trades with your husband. If your little darlings are up and at 'em at 5:30 A.M. no matter how late they're tucked in, it's better to make an every-other-day deal with your husband than an "I'll get up with them on weekdays if you do the weekends" arrangement. I don't have any science to back it up—just the fact that many mothers specifically suggested this. "It's much, much easier for me to get up at six with some semblance of good cheer when I know that tomorrow morning it's his turn," one of them put it. "If you're just living for the weekend, when you can sleep in—well, on Tuesday at 6 A.M., Saturday seems a million miles away."

If you can't get the quantity of sleep you need, at least try to improve the quality. Scientists break the sleep cycle down into stages. The deepest, most restful sleep is found in stages three and four. To get there and to stay there long enough to get its restorative qualities, you need to make your sleep conditions as optimum as possible. Some suggestions:

1. Limit your caffeine intake. "I'm not saying people need to cut out caffeine entirely," said Erman, "but if you're

having trouble falling asleep or staying asleep, start by cutting back in the afternoon and evening hours." Make it a rule for yourself: no coffee, cola, tea, or chocolate after dinner. Or even after 3 P.M.

Incidentally, if you're using caffeine as an antidote to fatigue, be aware that, while it will in fact perk you up, it's only a short-term remedy. When it wears off after a few hours you'll feel even more exhausted. And if you keep pouring it on, you risk caffeine overload, which can make you feel jittery and also make your sleep-deprivation crankiness worse.

2. Cut back on alcohol. Erman said alcohol does make it easier to fall asleep. "But it also tends to make sleep lighter throughout the rest of the night," he said.

3. Get regular exercise to ensure that your body will be as tired as your mind is at night. But get it done as early in the day as possible, certainly before dinner, Erman suggested. Otherwise, no matter how tired you are, you might be too revved up to fall asleep.

4. Make your sleep environment as restful as possible. Keep the bedroom dark, quiet, and at a comfortable temperature (most people sleep best when the room is between 60 and 65 degrees). Turn off the ringer on your bedside phone. Ask friends not to call or come by after, say, 10 P.M. Strive to keep external noises, such as a police siren or the beep of a car horn, out of the bedroom. Put in double-paned windows, for example. Erman said external noises don't have to wake you up in order to disrupt your sleep. Such noises can kick you out of a deep stage of sleep and into a less restful one. (And interestingly, though dream researchers say an external noise can't spark a dream, it can alter the course of one that's already in

progress. There you are, for example, walking down the aisle of your old college chemistry class, clad in nothing but your underwear, when suddenly your professor starts barking like a dog!)

Is the Sleep of Mothers Different?

Lots of women swear that no matter how optimum the sleep conditions, no matter how quiet the room or how silent the child, once we're mothers we never again sleep quite as soundly as we did prepregnancy, because we sleep with one ear cocked for that troubled "Mommy?"

Does motherhood, in fact, push most of us into the "light sleeper" category? And if so, is this a phenomenon of nature or nurture? I remember reading somewhere that the hours of insomnia that most women suffer in their final weeks of pregnancy are nature's way of preparing us for the sleepless nights to come. Is "Lite Sleep" another of Mother Nature's products for her fellow mothers?

Neurologist Shafor said she knows of no clinical studies documenting that women's sleep quality declines after childbirth. But she does say that she and her fellow sleep researchers have heard enough reports from mothers to confirm that the phenomenon is extremely common if not universal. She believes that the major cause of lighter maternal sleep is the higher anxiety level a woman has once she has borne a child and assumes the awesome responsibility of the well-being of another human being. This anxiety, of course, has psychological roots in the whole complicated bonding process. But according to Shafor, it also is probably due at least in part to the hormonal changes that accompany pregnancy and childbirth, which would explain why the most concerned and involved dads are often able to snooze on peacefully through even the most ear-splitting wails.

But Shafor believes some cases of lighter maternal sleep are primarily the result of physical problems incurred during pregnancy and childbirth (another logical reason the sleep of new dads is nowhere nearly as affected as that of their wives). One common postpartum sleep problem she sees in her sleep lab, for example, is something called restless legs syndrome. It's a malady suffered by many pregnant women in which they need to move their legs almost constantly; they just can't seem to find a comfortable position for them, especially while lying down. "Many pregnant women can get relief only by getting out of bed and walking around," Shafor said. Her theory is that the condition is caused by a change in the curvature of the spine during pregnancy as the fetus puts pressure on the area, particularly when the mother is lying on her back. Shafor said the problem can remain even after childbirth. "The symptoms may have decreased to the point where the woman no longer feels she has the syndrome, and yet her muscles are still sending 'restless' messages to the brain, which in turn disrupts the sleep," Shafor said. "She may wake up feeling fatigued or achy and not understand why."

Postpregnancy bladder problems also frequently affect the quality of sleep. It's difficult for the brain to relax enough to sink into the deeper levels of sleep when the bladder is sending "you have to go" messages.

Shafor said lighter sleep may also be the result of habits you've gained since pregnancy and childbirth that you've programmed into your biological clock. Let's go back to the bladder for example. In the last few weeks of pregnancy, most women become accustomed to having to get up a few times a night because the bladder is incapable of holding more than a few teaspoonfuls of urine. This get-up-and-go habit may become more deeply ingrained after birth, since you're having to get up for feedings anyway. In the end, long after your child is sleeping through the night and even if nocturnal visits to the bathroom are no longer physically necessary, your brain may still be programmed to avoid deep sleep so that it can wake you up to go, as usual.

Poor maternal sleep that's related to biological clock programming can usually be resolved with the help of a sleep specialist, according to Shafor. ("Although I just deprogrammed myself," said a mother who was tired of getting up twice a night to go to the bathroom. "I just said, 'Forget it!' and rolled over whenever I woke up and considered going. I guess my brain, and my bladder, finally got the message. I don't wake up for that anymore.") Shafor said there are also medications and other professional interventions available if your light sleep is primarily the result of a physical problem (and oftentimes you need to spend a night in a sleep lab for such a condition to be diagnosed as sleep disruptive).

But if your lighter sleep is the result of natural maternal anxiety (and that's the case for most of us), Shafor said there's little you can do but strive to improve the conditions affecting sleep quality that you can change: caffeine consumption, room temperature, and so on. She did add that mothers' anxiety levels tend to decrease as time goes by and we gain faith both in our ability to care for our children and in the strength and resiliency of their bodies and minds. Yes, they do make it through the night in one piece, and they do learn to calm themselves back to sleep from a nightmare, often before we can even reach their bedsides. I know that my own sleep got a little more sound after

Madeline turned seven months old, because I had read that that's the age when the incidence of sudden infant death syndrome drops off dramatically.

But, I worriedly asked Shafor, does the anxiety ever really diminish enough to give us even a semblance of our old, restful-before-children sleep? I told her that I've talked to several women in their late fifties and sixties who say that they still sleep poorly, even though their kids have long since left the nest. Are some of us doomed to be light sleepers for the rest of our lives? Shafor said that the poor sleep of these women is far more likely to be linked to the continuation of "light sleeper" habits—playing the radio all night, keeping a light on, or making bathroom trips—than to anxiety. But the most likely culprit, Shafor said, is age. Most people are unaware that we simply don't sleep as long or as deeply in our senior years, nor do we need to.

Let's hope that, for most of us, there will be a couple of good, restful years in there between the time Mother Nature reduces our nighttime maternal anxiety to almost nothing and Father Time decides that we're "seniors." Something to look forward to!

CHAPTER FIVE

CLAIMING YOUR NEW SEXUAL SELF

My friend Nonnie told me that about three weeks after she had her baby, she picked up a magazine that quoted a Masters and Johnson study that showed that many women resume having sexual intercourse within three weeks of childbirth. "I was stunned," she told me. "At that point I was about as interested in having sex as I was in driving a dogsled across the Arctic. In fact, I felt that way the whole first year."

At the other end of the spectrum, another friend, Linda, told me she enthusiastically resumed her sex life two weeks after delivery. "My doctor told us to abstain for six weeks before birth and for six weeks after," she said. "That's three months. No way! We figured as long as it didn't hurt me, it was okay. And it *didn't* hurt; I hadn't had an episiotomy." I asked Linda about lochia: didn't she still have it at two weeks postpartum? She nodded. "I just put my diaphragm in. It stopped the flow just like it does when I'm on my period."

Wondering which one of these women is more represen-
tative of the majority of postpartum women? Nonnie, no
contest. According to surveys much more recent than the
one taken by Masters and Johnson (in 1963!)—including
my own informal survey—most women do not resume sex
right away; and once they do resume sex they have it much
less often than they did prepregnancy.

According to a 1992 survey taken by L.A. *Parent* magazine, the percentage of couples who made love more than
three times a week plunged from 54 percent prekids to 5
percent postkids. In a similar 1988 *Parenting* magazine
survey, 34 percent of female respondents agreed with the
statement "Since I became a parent, sex is not as much fun
as it used to be," while another 20 percent went with
"Since I became a parent, sex is something from my
former life." Furthermore, a parent's altered sex life can
last not just for months but for *years*. Lots of people who
took part in both of these surveys were the parents of
toddlers and preschoolers, not infants. Marilyn Kentz—
who's one half of the comedy team known as "The Mommies" and whose youngest child is seven—sets female
audiences howling, according to *People*, when she comes
out on stage in a sexy, low-cut nightgown to talk about her
"favorite fantasy"—a shopping trip in which her kids behave.

Safe Sex

Before we get into why sex diminishes after a child is born
and what you can do if you (or your husband) are unhappy
with this state of affairs, let me address women who *are*
ready, willing, and eager to resume intercourse (who can
then skip all the rest of this chapter and go on to the next).
When is it safe to do so? This is another one of those

postpartum areas fraught with conflicting advice. Many physicians still routinely advise new mothers to wait a full six weeks in order to prevent infection in the recovering reproductive organs; others insist that this rule was written before antibiotics were available. Another rule of thumb you might hear is "You only have to wait till the lochia stops flowing." But in some women, the lochia flows for a full six weeks anyway. The best advice I heard was from gynecologist Neysa Whiteman: instead of waiting the usual six weeks for your postpartum checkup, have your doctor examine you as soon as you feel ready to resume sex. She says many women are completely healed and get the go-ahead at four weeks.

Temporary Physical Obstacles to Good Sex

There are a number of physical reasons in the first several months after childbirth that sex just may not feel as good as it used to. In the 1989 St. Paul, Minnesota, study of changes in women's physical health during the first postpartum year, researchers found that at three months 40 percent of new mothers had at least one complaint related to sexual function: discomfort with intercourse, decreased desire, and/or difficulty reaching orgasm. Even one year after delivery, a fifth of the mothers continued to have sexual problems. Here are some of the specific physical problems new mothers encounter.

Vaginal changes. Vaginal dryness and thinning of the vaginal walls can be blamed on the fact that estrogen levels plummet after childbirth, and estrogen is what helps vaginal cells lubricate. Your estrogen level stays low if you breastfeed, so nursing mothers may have to contend with vaginal problems for months.

Lack of desire. Many experts believe that the hormone mixture after childbirth, especially if you breastfeed, suppresses sexual desire and can make orgasm more difficult (or impossible) to achieve. "When you're nursing, you're in a semimenopausal state," said Scottsdale, Arizona, obstetrician and gynecologist (OB/GYN) Deborah Nemiro. "This is because prolactin, the hormone responsible for the production of breast milk, actually suppresses some of the other hormones so that you're essentially asexual. You do not have the urge for sex. In a lot of societies, sex is taboo as long as a woman is nursing. And that's probably not a bad idea since a nursing woman is dry and without desire."

On the other hand, Tracy Hotchner, who wrote the venerable reference *Pregnancy & Childbirth*, believes that many nursing women experience more intense or frequent orgasms. "The [nursing] hormones enlarge your veins and promote growth of new blood vessels in your pelvis," she wrote. "This raises the response potential of your vagina and clitoris."

Perhaps the middle ground here is that you may not have any sexual desire, but if you do end up having an orgasm, it's a whopper.

Sore perineum. It takes weeks for an episiotomy to heal, and two mothers told me that even after they believed they were completely healed they got a surprise—pain—at the height of passion. To avoid this situation, it's wise to monitor the healing of your episiotomy. You'll get a pretty good idea of whether the area will hurt during intercourse by pressing on the vaginal opening with your fingers.

One woman told me it was her husband who felt sexually inhibited by her episiotomy, which he had seen the doctor perform. "He was afraid of hurting me long after that area stopped hurting," she said. "He had been real nervous about having sex while I was pregnant, too. He had this crazy idea that the baby inside my uterus could somehow *see* what we were doing! So we had sexual problems for a long time!"

Breast discomfort. If you're nursing, physical arousal of the breasts during sex can give you an uncomfortable, engorged feeling. Some mothers (and fathers) may also be put off or embarrassed by the leaking or even spurting of milk when the mother is aroused. You may also simply dislike having your husband use your breasts for sexual pleasure while they are serving a more functional purpose, the nourishment of your child.

In a 1989 article in *Parenting* magazine about mothers and sex, two women said that their breasts lost all excitability for a long time after childbirth. "If I did not look down and see my husband on my nipple," said one, "I literally would not know that another person was in the room. I can't feel a thing." Said the other, "I think it just takes a long time. It took about 2½ to 3 years [for my breasts] to feel normal, and then I got pregnant again."

Being "touched out." Some women get all the physical intimacy they need and want just by mothering an infant, especially if they're breastfeeding. "When I'm not nursing my baby or 'wearing' her in a front pack, I've got my two-year-old battling for my lap," one mother told me. "When my husband comes home in the evening, what I want is a *break* from all that touch overload, not yet another person pawing at my body."

Fatigue/lack of sleep. It's hard to work up much enthusiasm for sex when you're reeling from fatigue, both the physical fatigue that results from lack of sleep and the mental kind that comes with the realization that you now have a twenty-four-hour-a-day responsibility. In fact, parents who participated in both the *L.A. Parent* and *Parenting* magazine sex surveys named being "too tired" as the number one reason their lovemaking had declined so much from prepregnancy days (and remember, many of these parents no longer have infants—their children are toddlers, preschoolers, or even older). Quipped one working mom who answered *Parenting* magazine's questions about sex: "Okay, but try not to wake me up while you're doing it." Said another, "I'd rather sleep than eat. I'd rather sleep than do anything."

Feeling "too loose." Often a woman's vaginal opening or vagina isn't as tight as it was prepregnancy, and this may decrease her own or her husband's physical sensations during intercourse.

High Anxiety

Many of the obstacles to good sex after you've had a baby have a psychological rather than a physical root.

Self-consciousness. Some women are embarrassed about, or their partners react negatively to, extra pounds or other differences in their postpartum bodies. This can lead to sexual inhibition in either or both parties. "I remember glancing at my husband while I was getting undressed one night, and the wistful look in his eyes clearly said, 'You don't look as good as you used to,' " I was told by a mother who is still battling to get rid of the fifty-five pounds she gained while pregnant. "Since then, I will not make love unless the lights are out."

Inhibited spontaneity. Many women have difficulty getting in the mood for sex because they always (even while sleeping) have an ear cocked toward the baby's room, listening for a possible cry. "It's like an automatic response. The split-second my husband touches me, our son—three rooms away—starts wailing," one mother complained to me. "It's like he has some kind of radar for detecting when I'm paying attention to someone besides him." (Incidentally, there's a theory that Mother Nature designed women to be more easily distracted during sex because in prehistoric times when a man was having sexual intercourse he was very vulnerable to prey, so that the woman had to be on alert.)

When children are older, many mothers—and fathers, too, for that matter—find their sexuality inhibited not by the possibility of a child's cry but by the possibility of her actual intrusion into the bedroom.

Fear of infection. Some women avoid sex because they fear it will give them an infection in their recovering reproductive organs. OB/GYN and *Parents* magazine columnist Sheldon Cherry has said that it reassures many women to know that if they haven't gotten an infection before the end of the initial healing phase (about a week after delivery), they're not likely to get one subsequently.

Fear of pregnancy. If you had a difficult childbirth, you may avoid sex for fear of getting pregnant and having to repeat the experience. I interviewed one mother who had had a thirty-three-hour labor and C-section. She said that even after three years she refuses to have sex during the seven days in the middle of her cycle despite the fact that her husband always uses condoms.

Another woman, the mother of a nine-month-old, told me that fear of pregnancy has made her sexually inhibited, as well, not because she had a difficult delivery but because she's terrified by the idea of having to take care of *two* helpless babies at once.

Resentment. Some women have trouble feeling loving toward their husbands because they believe these men are not giving them enough help, support, credit, or sympathy. Said one mother: "He did not spend nine months throwing up. He did not have his stomach cut open. He did not have to quit his job. He does not spend all day coping with poop and spit-up. His life barely changed at all, so neither have his sexual demands. He needs to just give me a break."

Inability to get out of the "Mommy mode." Many new mothers are so caught up in parenting tasks and their feelings for the baby are so overwhelming that they have difficulty making the psychological leap from nurturing mother to erotic wife. And this problem isn't limited to women, either: some fathers also have trouble seeing a mother as a sexual being. Sometimes a new father "connects maternity with his own mother, and it seems inconsistent with sexuality" is the way Boston psychologist Ron Levant once put it in *American Baby* magazine. Elvis Presley was one such father, his ex-wife, Priscilla, wrote in her autobiography. She said this was their major marital problem after daughter Lisa Marie was born.

Other paternal hangups. Fathers may avoid sex for other reasons. A study conducted by Sam Janus, Ph.D., a clinical associate professor of psychology at New York Medical College in Valhalla, New York, found that almost 30 percent of new fathers who actually witnessed the birth of the child later experienced some degree of impotence. I shared this statistic with two fathers, and both nodded as if to include themselves in that number. I asked them what they found so unsettling about watching the birth process. Said one (out of his wife's hearing): "Seeing all those organs so swollen and gaping made me feel like I never wanted to be down there again." (Of course, he has since gotten over that!) Said the other: "For me, it wasn't so much feeling grossed out as feeling guilty. I remember thinking to myself when I saw the baby's head crown 'That's what all that equipment is for—not for your personal enjoyment.'"

In a 1993 newspaper column, Dr. Joyce Brothers talked about another reason men sometimes have sexual problems after childbirth. A brand-new mother had written to Brothers commenting on the fact that so many men in her neighborhood seemed turned off about sex with their wives after the babies came, and started cheating on those wives. Brothers responded that this is most apt to happen when husbands feel shut out by wives, wives who suddenly seem interested only in the children. "This is one of many reasons husbands should be included in nurturing babies," Brothers wrote. "When husbands are actively involved with new babies, they bond with them faster, identify more with the difficulties and joys of parenting, and are less likely to have sexual problems after the baby arrives."

Getting Back Your Sexy Self

If you're unhappy with your sex life—you don't like sex anymore, aren't getting enough, or your husband wants more than you do—here are some things that can help.

Physical Remedies

Try artificial lubrication. Most postpartum women, especially those who are breastfeeding, produce little lubrication even when they're aroused, because of their low estrogen levels. A water-based lubricating product can alleviate this problem completely. "There should be a holiday to honor whoever invented K-Y jelly," one mother enthused to me. "I cannot sing its praises highly enough. It feels *exactly* like the real thing; and it's even better than the real thing because you can control the amount."

Another woman told me that the only problem she had with the lubricant was that it took her three days to psyche herself up to buy it. "Buying K-Y jelly is even more embarrassing than buying condoms or contraceptive foam," she said with a laugh. "When you buy those, you're announcing to everyone in the checkout line behind you 'I have sex.' When you buy a lubricant, everyone knows not only that you have sex but that you also have sexual problems." This woman went on to say that when she finally got up the nerve to buy lubricant, she bought three huge tubes of it, enough to last years. She doubled over laughing at the memory: "I believed people would think 'No one needs that much for sex. She must be buying it for a craft project or something.'" Incidentally, the investment was worth every penny, she said.

Warning: make sure the lubricant you buy is oil-free. Petroleum-based products (such as Vaseline) not only can weaken condoms and cause them to tear, they can also build up on the vaginal wall, which can disguise symptoms of an infection and cause other problems.

Experiment with positions. Remember reading in mags like *Cosmo* in your prebaby days that the woman-on-top position gives you the most control in regard to orgasm? Well, in your postbaby days, that position will also give you the most control over perineal pain, if you're still having it. One woman told me that she also found the "spoon" position—both of you on your sides, with the man in back—much more comfortable than the traditional missionary position. Try these—or experiment to find your own more comfortable sexual positions.

Tighten up. If you feel as if your vaginal opening or vagina is looser than it was prepregnancy and the physical sensations of intercourse aren't as pleasurable (or if that's your partner's complaint), Kegel exercises often result in great improvement (see "Tighten Up: K Power!" in Chapter 3).

Ensure your privacy. Once your child is able to climb out of the crib, get a lock for your bedroom door. An interesting alternative: Grease the outside doorknob with petroleum jelly. It's also a good idea to teach a child, right from the start, that a closed door means that one knocks and then waits for a response before entering. Don't feel guilty about taking these measures: they are vital for the health of your marriage.

If, despite your best efforts, your child does walk in on you, there's no need to run straight to a child psychiatrist. To reassure other mothers, one woman told *Parenting* magazine that while she was having sexual intercourse one night, her four-year-old evidently came into the bedroom undetected—and said the next morning, "You know, Mommy, if you play in your bed so hard you're going to break the springs." Said the mother, "So you see, she was not traumatized by our lovemaking; all she thought we were doing was wrestling around."

Be low key. You do not have to take this opportunity to educate your child about the birds and bees. Sexual intercourse is way too advanced a concept for most preschoolers to comprehend. Explaining that grownups who love each other simply like to wrestle and hug probably will suffice. If your child seems concerned that your partner was hurting you, reassure her that he wasn't and that you were having fun.

Take time for yourself. Spend some time absolutely and totally alone each day, even if it's only fifteen minutes or a half-hour. The best time: right after your child goes to bed. This break gives you a chance to change gears from your role as a mother to your role as a woman. Take a long bath, or read the paper, or do some stretching in front of the TV, or give yourself a pedicure. "This may seem like the opposite of intimacy," Los Angeles psychologist Stella Resnick said to the *L.A. Parent* sex survey participants, "but if you don't have some time to yourself, you'll take it when you're *with* the other person."

Attitude Adjustments

Work on your self-image. If you're feeling fat, flabby, or floppy, see Chapter 3 for tips on improving your physical condition and Chapter 10 for improving the way you see yourself.

Expect your husband, too, to go through a period of adjusting to your postbaby body. However, if his negative feelings continue for more than a few months, consider marriage counseling because his attitude may indicate that there's a more serious problem with the relationship (also see "Inability to Get Out of the 'Mommy Mode'" and "Other Paternal Hangups" above). One mother told me that despite her husband's assurances that she looked great, she really didn't believe him or feel desirable again until she went back to work 4½ months postpartum and found that *other* men obviously still found her desirable because they wanted to flirt with her.

Focus on quality, not quantity. "Many people think they're failures when they work hard all day and then don't feel like making mad, passionate love every night," Helen Singer Kaplan, director of the human sexuality program at New York Hospital–Cornell Medical Center, said in *Parenting*. "This is an unrealistic and destructive expectation." Kaplan advises couples to be far more concerned with the quality of the sex: when you do have it, make it really good.

Try to view sex as replenishment. Said Resnick in *L.A. Parent*: "If you're always feeling too tired or too busy [for sex]—the most popular complaints—that means you're running on reserves and draining your energy. Think of sex as valuable; physical contact is a way to de-stress, not just another requirement to fit into the day."

And according to *Redbook*, sex can do more than just relieve stress. Studies have shown that having regular, satisfying sex may also strengthen the immune system; that lovemaking is a remarkable sedative and helps to relieve insomnia; and that orgasm is a natural analgesic, relieving everyday aches and pains plus some PMS symptoms (see "PMS Busters" in Chapter 3). Added bonus: A 120-pound woman can burn up to eight calories a minute during sex.

It Takes Two

De-emphasize intercourse. If you're feeling guilty about your decreased sexual appetite and/or your diminished frequency of intercourse, there are plenty of ways to maintain physical intimacy with your partner without going all the way. Try eroticizing the mundane—for example, French-kiss your husband instead of pecking his cheek when you part in the morning. As a bonus, sex experts say that when you don't complete each contact with orgasm, you build up your appetite for sex.

Date your husband. Sexual sparks will be few and far between if you only view each other as Mommy and Daddy. You need regular time alone with your spouse— without interruption—to rekindle the old man-woman connection. Too overwhelmed to organize such dates? Make that *his* job. Or simply arrange for a sitter to come on a standing basis, say every Friday night, and just go to the same tacky but romantic Italian joint around the corner. Make it a rule that you cannot discuss your children or household problems. One mother, who quit a high-powered bank job to stay home during her baby's first two years, told me she subscribed to and always made time to read *People* and the *Wall Street Journal* so she'd have something not home-related to talk about with her husband.

Keep the lines of communication open. You shouldn't talk about children or household problems on your dates. But that doesn't mean you should *never* discuss such issues. In fact, both of you should clear the air on a regular basis. As psychologist Evelyn Bassoff once put it in *Parents* magazine, "Grievances between partners that are not talked out over the kitchen table have a way of sneaking into the bedroom." For best results, try couching complaints in "I" terms rather than as accusations—for example, "I need more help around the house" instead of "You don't do *anything* around here!"

It's also a good idea to share your feelings about sexual problems. One mom of a six-month-old told me that she finally admitted to her husband that she felt he wasn't initiating sex as often as he used to because he was turned off by her postbaby body. It turned out his sexual interest had diminished only because he, too, felt exhausted by his new responsibilities.

You may wish to share with your husband the information in the beginning of this chapter about the various reasons new mothers usually aren't very interested in sex. In his book *Confessions of a Pregnant Father*, writer Dan Greenburg lamented that nobody ever tells you this stuff. "Why do obstetricians and the guidebooks imply that you'll be having sex right up to the time you're fully dilated and that the longest it ever takes any normal couple to get back to regular sex is six weeks? If there could be a bit more candor in this area, new parents might feel they were within the mainstream of human experience rather than candidates for the Masters and Johnson Clinic."

One mother I know went out of her way to let her husband know that her lack of desire had nothing to do with him personally. "I told him that even if John F. Kennedy, Jr., were to burst through our front door wearing nothing but a loin cloth and panting for sex with me, I'd simply hand him the baby and ask him to watch her while I took a nap."

Forget about trying to have sex at bedtime. Though bedtime is the traditional time for having sex, it's the *worst* time for most parents. It is positively normal, especially in the first two years of parenthood, to be much more desirous of sleep than of sex at the end of a long day. Take the pressure off of yourselves and consider this much better choice: Naptime on Saturday or Sunday afternoon. If your child has given up naps, perhaps you could take him to a babysitter's house on one of those weekend afternoons and have your date with your husband then, at home. Anyway, it's much easier to get a babysitter on a Saturday afternoon than for a Saturday night.

Ask your husband for more help. Most of us have seen the statistics about just how much of the home management and childcare workload women are still shouldering despite the fact that the majority are also working outside the home. You may also have read articles, or voiced complaints yourself, about just how difficult it is to get a husband to do more. (Read more about this in Chapter 8.) If you find you're always too exhausted to want sex, however, the promise of more sex in exchange for more help can evidently be very effective. "I told my husband that if he would let me have every Saturday afternoon off by taking care of the kids, I might feel more energetic and romantic on Saturday night," my friend Nonnie told me. "We discovered I was right. This has worked like a charm for us."

Try erotica. Wait! Don't skip this section if you saw your first and last porn movie in college, venturing into one of those scuzzy downtown theaters with your boyfriend in an effort to show how bohemian/hedonistic/liberated/unshockable you were. It's true: traditional porn flicks are not the average woman's cup of tea. As one of my friends put it, "All you ever see are actresses performing, after begging to do so, sex acts that aren't exactly first on your basic woman's list of favorite sexual practices." Lynn Snowden, in a hilarious *Cosmo* piece, gave another reason that most women are turned off (instead of on) by porn: "It's the simple fact that male porn stars are either unbelievably sleezy looking, stone ugly, or both. The steroid freaks! The paunches! The bad skin, Brillo hair, unruly mustaches! There are times when a man appears on screen and you realize you dread the moment you'll see him nude, let alone *having sex* with someone." The bottom line about traditional porn flicks is this: these films are made by men for men.

In the last few years, however, savvy producers (many of them women) have begun to make soft-core porn films—"erotica" is the more genteel name for the category—especially for women. These films are a sort of hybrid of the romance novel and the traditional porn flick: they obviously are more visual than the novel, and there's less submissiveness and more plot, character development, sensuousness, and foreplay than in male-targeted porn. "And few if any blow jobs," a new mother told me quite candidly. "If you haven't been in the adult section of a video store since 1983," she continued, "I highly recommend that you duck into one soon. These films absolutely saved my sex life, if not my marriage. Believe me, your husband will enjoy them, too; there's lots of skin and lingerie." She said that if you can't identify an erotic film directed at women by its title or by other descriptive information on the cassette case, the name of the production company can be a clue. The companies catering to women often have feminine names (Tigress, Blush, and Femme are examples).

You may not even have to duck into the adult section of the video store if you have cable. As I write this, there is a very talked-about, steamy, and popular program late Saturday night on Showtime called "Zalman King's Red Shoe

Diaries." The series, guest-starring such mainstream actors as Ally Sheedy, is devoted entirely to female sexual fantasies and is targeted at female viewers. I have also seen erotica made for women and available by mail order advertised in the back pages of magazines such as *Cosmo.*

Consult an expert. If none of these suggestions helps and your sexual problems are causing a rift, some help from a professional will be an excellent investment. Your OB/ GYN will probably be your best resource for solving physical problems. I know three women whose doctors turned around their sex lives by fixing their episiotomies.

Your regular doctor may not be the right person to see, however. This was true for Dani, one mother I interviewed. She was having pain inside her vagina during intercourse 3½ months after birth and told me that she finally got around her embarrassment about talking about sex with her grandfatherly doctor by simply telling him that it hurt to wear a tampon. "Seconds later, I realized that only a few minutes earlier I'd told him I hadn't got my periods back yet," Dani said. "And I guess that dawned on him at the same time, because his face got even redder than mine as he figured out what I really meant. At any rate, his discomfort convinced me that he was not the right person to ask about my *other* sexual problem: the fact that I just never wanted sex, *period,* that I was only doing it for my husband's sake, and that this was making him very angry."

Dani is one of many mothers who would benefit by seeing a sex therapist with her husband. But when I advised her to seek such counseling she was horrified: Thanks to some magazine article she'd read back in the 1970s, she thought what a sex therapist did was serve as a surrogate for husband or wife in bed in order to resolve the problems. This kind of therapy is extremely rare; the major role of a sex therapist is to help couples discuss their sexual problems and then give specific suggestions for resolving those problems. (And you can rest assured that *these* folks won't be embarrassed by anything you tell them. All they hear about all the livelong day is sex, sex, sex.)

Your doctor or local medical school can give you a referral for a certified sex therapist. Or call the American Association of Sex Educators, Counselors, and Therapists at (312) 644-0828. That organization has listings for certified sex therapists nationwide.

Let's leave the subject of sex with a couple of upbeat thoughts. First, while the 1988 *Parenting* magazine survey I've mentioned frequently in this chapter found that sex is down among parents, it also found that *love* is up: four in ten of the new mothers who participated in the survey and 55 percent of the new fathers reported that they were more in love with their partner than ever. "I remember one night as I watched my husband so carefully bathing our baby, I kept thinking that this man had helped me create this incredible little person, and my eyes overflowed with tears of gratitude, and my heart overflowed with love for him," a friend told me. You and your husband have created the most powerful bond in the universe: your child.

Second, "eventually, life goes back to normal—pain disappears, exhaustion diminishes, sexual desire returns," wrote Carin Rubinstein, the Ph.D. who interpreted the sex survey for *Parenting*. Sex is a natural appetite, she quotes sex expert Masters, and simply needs to be stimulated after a period of abstinence.

Finally, keep in mind that *nobody is counting!* If you and your mate are both happy with your sex life, it doesn't matter how often you "do it."

CHAPTER SIX

So Nice, I'll Do It Twice

Thinking about a Second Baby

A couple I know who had mixed feelings about having a second child finally sat down and made a pro and con list. While the pro list ended up significantly longer than the con, the couple still had their doubts. "We finally just decided to let Mother Nature decide," the female half of that couple told me. "We stopped using birth control, but we didn't go out of our way to have intercourse near my ovulation, as we had for our first child. We just had sex whenever we felt like it—make that whenever we felt up to it." Mother Nature did decide. This couple now has a four-year-old son and a nine-month-old daughter.

If you, too, are on the fence about having a second baby or if you've already decided you want another one, this chapter will tell you what you can expect physically—how a second pregnancy and delivery differ from the first. And I will offer some defensive strategies to try, the second time around, in order to minimize pregnancy's negative effects on your body. (You'll find information about the long-term physical effects, both good and not so good, of bearing more than one child sprinkled throughout Chapter 2. And how a second child changes a family's everyday life is discussed in Chapter 8.)

Is It Easier to Conceive a Second Child?

Evidently, the answer to that question appears to be yes, at least for one big group of people: those who had trouble getting pregnant the first time. Deborah Nemiro, M.D., a Scottsdale, Arizona, obstetrician and gynecologist, told me that OB/GYNs talk about this phenomenon all the time. A long-infertile woman will go through an infertility workup and some kind of treatment, will finally get pregnant and deliver her first child, and then—boom!—will easily get pregnant without help a second time. She said this is frequently true not only of women with specific infertility causes such as endometriosis (see the section on this condition in Chapter 2) but also in cases where doctors simply can't pinpoint a reason for a couple's inability to conceive.

My own parents fall into this latter category. It took them six frustrating years to conceive their first child, my oldest sister, and my mother's doctor couldn't come up with any reason for the infertility (keep in mind, however, that this was in the "ancient" 1950s). But within five years of Barbara's birth, my mother conceived and gave birth to three more children.

Why does this happen? Nemiro can only speculate. During pregnancy, she said, the placenta makes a lot of estrogen and progesterone to suppress the usual female cycle. Perhaps this suppression causes the system to bounce back stronger—and consequently more fertile— after childbirth.

This is not, however, the case with every couple who has already had a child. In fact, if you've ever heard the statistic that one in twelve couples in the U.S. is unable to get pregnant, you may be surprised to know that half of these couples have already conceived (often with little or no difficulty) and given birth to at least one baby or have suffered a miscarriage. This condition is called secondary infertility.

The causes of secondary infertility are just about the same as the causes of primary infertility. And couples with secondary infertility grapple with the same anguish and frustration, with one difference: they often feel (or others make them feel) as if they have no right to complain. "I can't tell you how many people have said things along the lines of 'Don't be so greedy. At least you have Jason,' " one mom told me. "These people have the audacity to say that, even though they have two or three children of their own. I've learned not to tell people about our problem. And when they ask, 'When are you guys going to produce a sister or brother for Jason?' (and they always do, though that's another thing that's none of their business), I just tell them we haven't decided yet whether to have a second child."

Often, secondary infertility is a result of the aging process. You may have conceived your first baby easily at age twenty-eight but have trouble at thirty-four. After thirty, the rate at which women conceive declines slowly but steadily. Experts believe men's fertility also declines—the quality of sperm and its fertilization ability apparently decrease starting at age forty-five. Another common, age-related condition that may cause infertility is fibroids, benign tumors in the uterus. This condition tends to strike women in their thirties and forties.

Experts urge couples with secondary infertility—or primary infertility, for that matter—to seek help after only six months of trying if the woman is over age thirty. The good news is that infertility experts can identify the cause of secondary infertility 90 percent of the time and can help the couple achieve another pregnancy in 75 percent of those cases.

What Will Be Different?

Morning sickness. Though we've all heard women say things like "I had morning sickness every single day for the first five months with each of my boys but none at all with my little girl" (or vice versa), on average a woman's experiences with nausea and morning sickness tend to repeat themselves from pregnancy to pregnancy. If even the *smell* of coffee gave you the dry heaves in your first pregnancy, for example, be prepared to gag as your husband perks his morning fix during your second pregnancy, too.

"Showing." Because the abdominal support structure will not be as strong as it was during the first pregnancy, you will "show" earlier than you did during the first go-around. If you started wearing maternity clothes in your fourth or fifth month the first time, don't be surprised if you have to haul them down from the attic in the third month of your second pregnancy.

Aches and pains. Less abdominal support, coupled with looser pelvic floor muscles, is also the reason second-timers have more pelvic ligament pains and more of a sense of pelvic pressure and heaviness than first-timers, according to Deborah Nemiro. "Basically, for some reason there are more aches and pains all over the body," said Nemiro, who has given birth to four babies of her own. "It's strange. For some of it there's an explanation, and for some of it there isn't."

Braxton Hicks contractions. Nemiro said looser conditions around the uterus and birth canal area are also probably responsible for the fact that women carrying second (or subsequent) babies have many more Braxton Hicks contractions (also sometimes called false labor pains) than women do in their first pregnancies.

Feeling movement. Many moms with two children told me that they felt their second babies kick or move much earlier than they felt the first. "It's because your uterus, which was stretched out the first time, is thinner the second time," one mother explained to me. Nemiro disputed that: "Actually, it's your abdominal wall musculature that's been stretched out a little bit," she said. "At any rate, I'm not sure if you can actually feel the baby kick earlier or if you're just more familiar with what that feels like. A lot of women in their first pregnancies will not recognize kicking until twenty-two weeks or so, and then they'll look back and say, 'Oh, so that's what that was.' Whereas a woman who has been pregnant before can recognize that sensation from the first twitch."

Physical annoyances. If you didn't get them fixed after the first time, annoyances such as hemorrhoids, varicose veins, and stress incontinence tend to worsen with each pregnancy. So do pregnancy backaches. Interestingly, the Melpomene Institute for Women's Health Research has found that backache during pregnancy seemingly has nothing to do with how much weight you gain or how much your baby weighs. Instead, they've seen (but haven't tried to explain) an association between back pain and maternal age and number of previous pregnancies.

"This may be because women aren't getting back into shape after they have their babies," said Doris Flood, a San Diego physical therapist who teaches a class on preventing and alleviating back pain during pregnancy (nine out of ten of her students are in their second or third pregnancies).

Obstetrical complications. One fairly common obstetrical complication, placenta previa, is more common in women who have already had a previous baby or two than in first-timers. Only 10 percent of pregnant women with this condition—in which the placenta has implanted low in the uterus, covering the opening—are first-time mothers, while mothers who have had four babies run a one in twenty risk of developing it with their fifth pregnancy.

Women who develop gestational diabetes (see Chapter 2) in their first pregnancy usually, but not always, get it again in subsequent pregnancies.

On the other hand, if you had toxemia (high blood pressure)—another common obstetrical complication—in your first pregnancy, your chance of developing it in the second is slight.

Length of pregnancy. Contrary to popular belief, women who have previously given birth tend to have slightly longer pregnancies than first-timers. But as a general rule, delivery timing is about the same from pregnancy to pregnancy. For example, if you were early the first time, you'll most likely go early the second. If your first pregnancy lasted more than forty-two weeks (which is considered "postterm" and is usually the point at which doctors want to intervene) your chances of going that long the second time are around 50 percent.

Engagement. In most first pregnancies, women experience what's called engagement, or lightening, a couple of weeks before labor starts. This is when the baby's head drops into the pelvis, which makes it easier for the mother to breathe but more difficult for her to walk. In second and subsequent pregnancies, engagement does not usually occur until labor actually begins.

Labor Is Faster, But . . .

In a 1992 *Parents* magazine survey of 72,000 mothers and their birth experiences, 65 percent of the women who had given birth more than once said the second birth was easier than the first. It's obvious that these women defined easier as *faster*—everyone knows that the average second labor is hours shorter than the first. (I am a second baby whose mother labored only forty-five minutes.)

What may come as a surprise to you, however, is that labor is actually more intensely painful for second-time mothers. In one of the studies that support this, labor and delivery nurse Nancy Lowe and colleagues at Ohio State University asked sixty-five first-time mothers and one hundred moms with more than one birth experience how painful labor was at various stages. The first-timers reported more pain during the initial stages of labor than did the veteran moms. But Lowe found the latter group of mothers experienced a very dramatic increase in pain in the final stages, as they were pushing the baby out.

What's happening here, according to both Lowe and Nemiro, is that, first of all, the cervix of the veteran mother dilates more rapidly. "The pain receptors in the cervix are related to stretch," Nemiro said, "and the faster the cervix dilates, the more painful it's going to be." Also, the birth canal "gives" more easily the second time around, enabling the baby to push through more quickly than in a first-time mother—a factor that intensifies pain.

"Why doesn't anyone tell you this?" a friend lamented. "I had an epidural with my first baby and went unmedicated with my second because everyone told me it would be a piece of cake. In retrospect, I should have done it the other way around." Two other moms told me that while Lamaze breathing techniques were somewhat helpful during their first labors, they weren't useful at all during the second. "It's harder to stay in control the second time around," Nemiro said.

Lowe told *Health* magazine she feels all pregnant women should be warned that their second birth won't be the same as their first. "If they understood that their labor would be more quick and intense during the late stages, they could handle it better," she said.

The good news, according to Nemiro, is that almost all veteran moms actually push the baby out in no time flat. "Many have to push just once or twice and the baby is propelled out by a contraction," she said. The experience of my friend Roberta is typical of most of the veteran moms I interviewed: it took her almost a half-hour to push out her first vaginally delivered baby; ninety seconds to push out the second.

If you're a mother who delivered by C-section the first time around, see "The Postcesarean Body" in Chapter 2 for more information about subsequent vaginal or cesarean births.

Postpartum for Veterans

Afterpains, contractions of the uterus as it returns to its prepregnancy size, tend to be worse after a second pregnancy in comparison to a first, and Nemiro said they get progressively worse with each subsequent pregnancy. The theory is that the uterus, having been stretched out yet again, has to work harder each time to regain its former tone.

The milk of second-time moms tends to come in a little earlier than it did the first time, and engorgement typically isn't as uncomfortable. "Engorgement the first time was hell, but it wasn't even a third as bad the second time," says Doris Flood, who has two young sons. "Why? I think your body becomes more efficient at the whole babymaking and nourishing process with each experience. I had much less leaking the second time, too. And I didn't have to pump so much."

On the other hand, veteran moms who nurse tend to have more bouts of mastitis (infection in a milk duct). Being stressed out or fatigued is believed to make women more prone to the problem, and dealing with both a newborn and a toddler or preschooler is certainly more stressful than caring for just the newborn alone.

If you developed postpartum depression after your first birth, you have a one in five chance of a repeat bout after your second. You have a fifty-fifty chance of getting postpartum psychosis after subsequent births if you suffered that disorder the first time around. (See Chapter 7 for more information about these conditions.)

If your second birth is an elective cesarean (perhaps because you had a cesarean the first time around), your recovery pain will be less than it was if you labored before your first such surgery.

Nemiro said it's generally harder to get your abdominal muscles back into shape after the second baby. My friend Kim will testify to that: "I actually gained less weight with my second baby but I had to work out more often and for a longer period of time in order to get my stomach flat again," she said.

Defensive Strategies

If you're planning to get pregnant again or you're in your early months of a second pregnancy (or a first pregnancy, for that matter), there are things you can do this time around to prevent or at least minimize the negative effects pregnancy and childbirth can have on the body.

Be strict about your weight gain. Keep your weight gain to less than thirty pounds. If you read Chapter 2, you know that excessive weight gain during pregnancy contributes to a host of postpartum problems, including a "loose" vagina and stress incontinence. The larger your baby, for example, the more stretching and trauma there will be in the pelvic region. In addition, excessive weight gain plays a role in both postpartum skin tone and stretch marks. How much weight you gain during pregnancy also affects how large your breasts get and, consequently, the postpartum sag factor. Researchers even believe that when a pregnant woman who is carrying a female fetus gains too much weight, she is increasing that *daughter*'s chances of later contracting breast cancer. And finally, according to OB/GYN Nemiro, "I see women do so much better in terms of regaining their self-esteem when they limit their weight gain to twenty-five to thirty pounds. The weight comes off in six weeks, and they feel somewhat like themselves again. They like their bodies again."

It's a good idea not only to limit your weight gain but to be careful about when you put those pounds on. If you put on too much of the weight too early in your pregnancy, it'll end up as fat you'll be battling to get rid of postpartum. "If you gain fifteen pounds in your first trimester [and] then limit your weight gain to three to four pounds a month for the rest of your pregnancy, you will be stuck with the extra weight," Anita Parnes La Sala, M.D., a specialist in maternal-fetal medicine and assistant clinical professor of obstetrics and gynecology at the Columbia University College of Physicians and Surgeons, told *Parents* magazine. She explained that this is because your caloric intake in the first trimester isn't shared with the baby, which is still in the embryonic stage. The placenta, which passes your nutrients on to the baby, isn't even formed yet.

Exercise. During pregnancy, regular exercise provides a variety of both physical and psychological benefits. It can help you keep your weight gain in check. It can ease or prevent backaches. It can help you fight fatigue. It can help you sleep better. It can make you feel better about yourself. It can actually improve your cardiovascular fitness. When you stay in good condition during your pregnancy, it's easier to lose weight after childbirth. And many in the medical community believe that regular exercise during pregnancy shortens labor and delivery.

A University of Vermont College of Medicine study found that women who exercise regularly during pregnancy not only have shorter labors, they also begin labor about five days earlier, have fewer cesarean sections, and deliver babies with less acute fetal stress than nonexercising pregnant women. The babies of the exercising women were also lower in weight—and that, said the researchers, "may actually turn out to be an advantage in terms of cardiovascular risk in later life."

Even the conservative American College of Obstetrics and Gynecology (ACOG) recommends that pregnant women get regular exercise, provided they have the approval of their physicians (because some obstetrical conditions such as high blood pressure make exercise off-limits). Overdoing it can divert oxygen and blood from the fetus, so ACOG has issued these specific guidelines about exercise and pregnancy:

• Your heart rate should not exceed 140 beats per minute. (How to tell: find your pulse at your neck, wrist, or chest and count the beats for six seconds; multiply by ten.) Gynecologist Whiteman's rule is you should be able to talk comfortably during exercise.

• A period of strenuous activity should not exceed fifteen minutes.

• After the fourth month, avoid any exercise that must be performed lying flat on your back, because the weight of the baby on your vena cava (heart vein) can impede your (and his) circulation.

• Don't hold your breath or strain.

• Make sure your caloric intake is adequate not just for your pregnancy but also for your exercise program (your doctor can help you with this).

• Your temperature while exercising should never exceed 100.4 degrees Fahrenheit.

Your hospital, local fitness center, and/or community college probably offer an exercise class for pregnant women. See "The Exercise Factor" in Chapter 3 for some advice on exercise videos and books.

Wear supportive bras. Wear a supportive, high-quality maternity bra and then a supportive, high-quality nursing bra. You may recall from Chapter 2 that some sagging after each pregnancy is inevitable. But you can save some of the elasticity of the ligaments supporting your breasts by wearing a good maternity bra during pregnancy and a good nursing bra during breastfeeding. They are different things, so don't try to get by with just buying a nursing bra for the whole pregnancy/breastfeeding period, because at least some of the time it won't fit you right or provide the support you need.

You can expect your breasts to grow by at least one back size and up to three cup sizes during your pregnancy. A maternity bra is designed to grow along with your expanding breasts and rib cage, but you'll need to buy a new, larger maternity bra at least once after your initial purchase to accommodate all the growth.

Don't buy your first nursing bra until the final weeks of your pregnancy. Make sure there's a finger's width of space between your breast and every area of the bra cup to allow room for growth (your breasts may increase yet another back size and cup size between your final weeks of pregnancy and your first week of nursing).

When buying both your maternity and nursing bras, keep these additional tips in mind:

• The bra should have wider-than-a-normal-bra straps (look for three-quarters of an inch to two inches) that are adjustable.

• The cups should cover the breasts entirely.

• The cup support should be comfortable. Rigid underwire can cause pain in breasts that are already swollen.

• Be sure you're buying the right back size. If the back of the bra rides up, the back size is probably too large. If the bra feels tight around your rib cage or you notice that the band fabric is crumpling or stretching, the back size is probably too small.

Use elastic stockings for varicose veins. If you go into pregnancy with varicose veins, wear elastic stockings (also called compression stockings). They can't stop new varicose veins from forming, but they can slow the process. They'll also make your legs feel better. And if you do get new varicose veins, the odds that they'll disappear after delivery are better if you wear this type of stocking (but you have to do so from the *beginning* of your pregnancy).

Wear supportive shoes. You can reduce the amount of permanent, pregnancy-related stretching and growth of your feet (see Chapter 2) by wearing sturdy shoes. Glenn Gastwirth, D.P.M., deputy executive director of the American Podiatric Medical Association, said your best bet is a shoe that laces up and that has a strong, rigid counter (the area of the shoe that surrounds the heel). The worst shoes to wear are the kind that are easiest for pregnant women to put on: thongs, slippers, and shoes that have no backs.

Stay out of the sun. You can prevent or at least minimize pregnancy-related skin pigment changes, such as the series of brownish stains across the face known as the mask of pregnancy, by limiting your sun exposure. "Women who get a lot of sun exposure during pregnancy are more prone to the mask, so you should wear a good sunscreen and preferably a hat, too, when you go out," said dermatologist Peter Rullan, M.D. He added that while most pigment changes clear up in the six months after delivery, some women need professional help to get rid of them.

Practice scrupulous dental hygiene. For many women, the lifelong battle against gum disease begins in pregnancy, when high hormonal levels allow gingivitis (an early stage of gum disease) to take hold and thrive (see Chapter 2). You can keep it under control by brushing and flossing religiously and getting regular professional cleanings throughout your pregnancy.

Be prepared for your heart to double in size. It's very common to worry that you could never love a second child as much as you love your first. Not to worry, according to every mother of two that I interviewed. "You fall in love with the second one just as hard," said my friend Rachel. "You have the same sense of overwhelming infatuation. In fact, you almost ache to spend more time with the second one because your life is so busy you never feel like you're getting enough."

Ann Pleshette Murphy, editor-in-chief of *Parents* (who has excellent taste in baby names), once offered her own experience as reassurance that a mother of two will, indeed, have enough love to go around: "Somehow my heart has miraculously expanded to embrace both of my children with equal intensity," she wrote. "What I feel for my newborn son has in no way depleted my love for Madeleine. In fact, as I watch her holding her brother and hear her say, 'His tiny fingers are so beautiful. And his cheeks are beautiful. He's a nice baby, Mama,' I am consumed with love for her and for the relationship she will have with her brother."

PART TWO:
SOUL

CHAPTER SEVEN

HAPPINESS AND HORMONES

The New Mother's Brain

A new mother grapples with so many psychological changes that instead of including a section called "Brain" in Chapter 2, I'm devoting several chapters to the subject. This one deals with emotional upheaval during the first postpartum year.

The Baby Blues

After your baby is born, your body will begin to reel from the massive drop in hormones that occurred upon delivery. Hormone levels actually drop tenfold, to levels so low that they would be considered abnormal in a woman who had not just given birth. One of the probable effects of this hormonal plunge, which usually happens about three or four days after birth, is a condition called the "baby blues." It is so common you will be in the minority if you *aren't* affected. The condition, which is exacerbated by the fatigue that comes from both sleep deprivation and (if this is your first) the psychological adjustment that must be made to a totally new lifestyle, usually manifests itself as sadness and weepiness. Mary Hart of "Entertainment Tonight" fame, for example, said that for the first two weeks after her son was born, she cried for no reason at all. "Flowers would arrive and I'd burst into tears," she told *Good Housekeeping.* "Someone would call about the baby and I'd cry. Even news stories on TV would make me cry."

Keep in mind, however, that the baby blues don't always mean melancholy. A handful of moms I interviewed said that they weren't weepy or sad at all, just irritable as hell. One mother even called the condition the "baby bitchies." "My son was a voracious nurser," she told me. "He wanted to eat every hour, and it left me exhausted. I remember one afternoon when he was about five days old and I was trying to nap. He started crying, and I just turned my back on the bassinet and said, 'Oh, shut up!' My husband walked into the bedroom and said, 'How can you tell an innocent baby to shut up?' And I screamed at him, 'You shut up, too!' "

In a similar but lighter vein, comedian Cathy Crimmins called her own postpartum bout with the baby blues "the perfect time to confront my mother about a favorite pair of socks that she shrank by mistake when I was in third grade," she wrote in her hilarious book, *Curse of the Mommy* (Putnam). "I also remember trying to clear the air by calling my husband at the office to confront him about something he did on our second date."

A couple of other mothers told me that they sank into funks of resentment and had thoughts like "I *hate* motherhood" or "Why did I ever want to do this?" or even "I'm going to put him up for adoption."

For one of my friends, the baby blues were characterized by anxiety instead of sadness. In the week after her baby was born, she kept having bizarre, graphic fantasies of her husband being killed by someone at his office or dying in a horrible car wreck on the way home. "I finally realized that I was just really anxious because I felt so dependent on him," she said. "Dependent on him not just to support us financially but to come home and relieve me of some of the responsibility of taking care of this completely helpless human being."

Such out-of-character feelings and behavior should subside within a couple of days or weeks, as your hormones return to normal levels (although don't be surprised if you go through a minibout with the blues when you stop breastfeeding, thanks again to hormones). Because of this, your best bet for coping is simply to keep telling yourself that "this, too, shall pass." Here's what else can help.

Try to get as much rest and sleep as you can. Fatigue and sleep deprivation worsen mood swings. Ask for help in keeping the household running those first few weeks. And force yourself to eat well and regularly; the drop in blood sugar that often occurs when a person hasn't eaten for a while can in itself produce irritability and depression.

Take a walk. Exercise is believed to trigger the release of endorphins, chemicals in the brain that boost your mood.

Don't forget your vitamins. Ask your doctor if you might take extra Vitamin B-6, which is often prescribed for depression.

Talk to other mothers. Go where you're likely to find other new moms: the park, postpartum exercise classes, hospital-sponsored parenting support groups. Even if the moms you meet no longer have newborns, they'll most likely remember and share some of the negative/panicky/

sad feelings they had during those difficult first weeks. This will help you understand how normal your feelings are.

Your husband may also provide a sympathetic or even *empathetic* ear. After all, though his hormones haven't gone bonkers, there have been major changes in his life, too. In fact, he also may be depressed. In one recent study, 62 percent of new fathers reported feeling "blue" at some point after the birth.

Write about your feelings. If you can't talk about your negative feelings, write them out. This is the advice James Pennebaker, Ph.D., a professor of psychology at Southern Methodist University, has for new mothers. He told *American Baby* magazine that in one of his recent studies, he found that students were helped when they wrote about traumas they had previously bottled up inside. (Added bonus: after the students had been writing a few days, Pennebaker said, their blood samples showed that their immune systems were healthier than before they had started writing.)

Cry. Feel like weeping? Then do it. There's an old Yiddish proverb that says, "Soap is to the body as tears are to the soul." And there just may be a scientific basis for the fact that almost everybody feels better after a good cry. Experts believe emotional tears may be a way for the body to get rid of stress-induced substances. Tears, it seems, contain certain hormones, such as prolactin, that are produced during stress.

Postpartum Depression (PPD)

PPD is a more serious mood disorder that can occur during the first postpartum year, and it affects almost 10 percent of new mothers. Some of its symptoms are similar to those of the baby blues: anxiety or panic, frequent crying, and/or fantasies of disaster are examples. Other symptoms are not similar, and these include insomnia, a desire to leave the family, loss of appetite, inability to make simple decisions, aversion to the baby, fear of harming the baby, overwhelming despondency, and loss of interest in previously pleasurable activities. However, the two major clues that you may be suffering postpartum depression instead of the simple baby blues are the onset and the duration. Instead of striking within days of birth as the baby blues do, PPD generally begins two to six weeks after delivery and can start at any time up to six months postpartum. PPD also lasts much longer than the baby blues. It may go on for months or even for the whole first year, and it often deepens as time passes.

Like the baby blues, PPD is believed to be triggered by the postpartum hormonal crash, but researchers believe that women who fall into full-blown postpartum depression also have one or more psychosocial and biological vulnerabilities to that condition. Some of these vulnerabilities include:

• A history of depression or previous PPD

• A history of hormonal problems such as PMS

• A family history of mood disorders

• A recent move

• A recent death in the family

• Marital problems, or having a husband who's away from home a lot

• A premature baby

- A pregnancy complication such as diabetes or placenta previa

- Being used to spending the majority of time outside the home

If you suspect you have PPD, it's important to seek help, both for your own mental health and the baby's. Experts say that in the first year of life a baby depends on interaction with her primary caregiver in order to learn about herself and her world, and a depressed mother may not be able to respond adequately. Some studies have found, in fact, that the children of mothers with PPD are more prone to developing emotional and behavioral problems themselves.

Sometimes a mother with PPD is hospitalized—with her baby, whenever possible. One mother I talked to told me that about three weeks after birth she became paranoid that she was going to accidentally kill her baby. She was afraid if she took his temperature, the thermometer would break inside him and cause him to bleed to death. She was afraid if she gave him a bath he'd accidentally drown. Finally, she couldn't even pick him up for fear of accidentally dropping him on his head. That's when her husband insisted she check into the hospital. She spent a week there.

PPD can be very successfully treated; don't feel that you are at its mercy because there's a hormonal component. Treatment generally consists of psychotherapy in conjunction with medication. Usually, that medication is a nonaddictive antidepressant drug, and some of the drugs in this class are okay for nursing mothers. Some doctors administer hormones. A few years ago, British researchers announced that they'd had great success in using Estraderm (the estrogen patch) to treat severe PPD cases. And Katharina Dalton, the PMS expert (read more about her and her theories in "PMS Busters" in Chapter 3), reports that she has helped new mothers at high risk of developing PPD avoid the condition altogether by administering progesterone right after the women deliver.

Doctors usually also advise women with PPD to join a support group of other mothers battling depression. These groups are often sponsored by local hospitals. If you don't know of one, you can get a referral to a group in your area by calling an organization called Depression After Delivery (DAD) at (800) 944-4773, or write to P.O. Box 1282, Morrisville, PA 19067. This organization was founded in 1985 by an art teacher who had a bout of severe postpartum psychosis (see below) that required her to be hospitalized, after which she lapsed into a six-month depression.

When you seek help for PPD, be sure that your doctor rules out any other physical problem that may be causing your depression. For example, researchers believe that as many as 11 percent of women suspected of having PPD actually have a temporary form of hypothyroidism called postpartum thyroiditis, in which an inflammation of the thyroid gland results in symptoms such as fatigue, lethargy, and forgetfulness, which are also common to depression. A simple blood test will reveal if this is the real problem. It can be easily and effectively treated with a thyroid medication.

Postpartum Psychosis

The most serious of the hormonally triggered postpartum mood disorders, postpartum psychosis, is also the most rare, affecting only about one in one thousand new mothers. Unlike PPD, which comes on gradually, postpartum psychosis hits very suddenly and is marked by a personality change, delusions, hallucinations, and a tendency toward violent behavior.

Susan Hickman, a San Diego psychotherapist and expert on postpartum psychosis, has said that a woman with this disorder often fluctuates between rationality and psychosis, all the while appearing completely normal. "It is very similar to dreaming while you are awake," Hickman told the *Los Angeles Times* on the eve of testifying for the defense in the case of a woman with the disorder who killed her baby. "Part of the reality that the mother is responding to is the real world and part of it is like a dream state where she sees things and hears things that other people don't."

We have all read tragic and horrifying examples of this in the newspaper: the mother who drowned her baby because she believed it had grown devil's horns; another who smothered her infant because a voice told her it was the only way to keep the earth from exploding into a million pieces.

England has for the past fifty years recognized postpartum psychosis as a cause in infanticides, and the maximum sentence for a mother who kills her baby in the first year of life is manslaughter. Even if the mother is convicted, she gets treatment, not prison. In 1989, California became the first U.S. state to enact legislation that recognizes postpartum psychosis, requiring a woman who is arrested for a violent crime and thought to be suffering from a postpartum mood disorder to be hospitalized for her protection and evaluated within twenty-four hours. (The latter requirement is important because in many cases of infanticide the woman is not examined for weeks, and by that time the psychotic episode may be over.) Despite this progress, most mothers who commit infanticide in the United States are not acquitted.

It should be stressed that not *all* women with postpartum psychosis go off the deep end. Hickman says only about 6 percent of affected women kill their babies or themselves. This disorder, too, is highly treatable, usually with hospitalization and antipsychotic drugs such as Thorazine, and most women recover fully within six months.

Of Human Bonding

A mother who had a very long and difficult labor that ended with a C-section told me that her baby blues were deepened by her belief that because she could not be with her newborn daughter for the first few hours after her birth, the "bond" between them would never be as strong as it could have been. "I had read that you must bond right after birth or you lose the opportunity forever," she said.

Scientists have done far more research about bonding between animal mothers and their babies than they have about humans. In fact, I was unable to even find a concise and semicoherent definition of this mysterious and powerful force that links mother and child for life. But enough human research has been conducted in the past few years so that you can stop worrying if, because of your own surgery, medical problems in the baby, or even hospital rules, you and your baby are separated for a few hours after birth. Researchers believe that *bonding is not limited to any one particular time*, that the bond is forged over a matter of weeks and months, not hours.

Television producer Diane English, creator of "Murphy Brown," decided to demonstrate just that in the now infamous episode in which Murphy finally gives birth. "There's a nice scene at the end where the nurse puts the baby in Murphy's arms and she doesn't know what the hell to do with it," English told the *Los Angeles Times* just before the episode aired. "Bonding is not something that naturally happens to women right away, and it certainly isn't happening to her. She doesn't know what to make of this child. She begins apologizing to it right away."

Most researchers believe that women who spend a lot of time with their babies right after birth do have a head start on forming an attachment; intriguingly, this may be thanks to physiological rather than psychological reasons. For example, some studies have suggested that a new mother's heightened sense of smell in the first couple of days after birth may help her bond with the baby. (How heightened? In one study, mothers were able to pick out their own babies from a group of them by smell alone only six hours after birth.)

Other research points to hormones as bond promoters in the first few hours after birth. For example, a University of Toronto study indicated that cortisol (a hormone released in a woman after she expels the placenta) creates "a state of arousal" in her that probably makes her more receptive to forging a bond. The results of animal studies have convinced some scientists that oxytocin (the hormone that causes the uterus to contract during labor) also may encourage bonding in human females, because one of its effects in animal mothers is to reduce fear and ease an animal's approach to her new offspring.

Still, to reiterate, a strong and lasting attachment *is not* dependent on the mother and baby spending a lot of postdelivery time together. Researchers believe the quality of the attachment is determined by a multitude of factors. One study that proves this was conducted by Herbert Leiderman, M.D., a professor of psychiatry and behavioral sciences at Stanford University. He studied mothers of full-term infants who took on the full-time care of their babies one to three days after birth and mothers of premature infants who had to spend two to three months, on average, separated from their babies after birth. Leiderman found that while the mothers of the preemies showed less commitment and self-confidence in the beginning, after only one month this was no longer the case. And by the time the babies were twenty-one months old, there was no difference in the maternal behavior of the mothers, except that the mothers of the preemies had *more* interaction with their toddlers than the full-term mothers.

In other research, Leiderman found that, among other things, the behavior of the baby and the socioeconomic status of the mother have a big effect on the progression and strength of the attachment. For example, a happy, smiling baby is easier to bond with than a colicky one because of the positive feelings the happy baby's behavior elicits in the mother. And the stress and worry that come with poverty can make it harder for an economically deprived mother to form a secure attachment with her child.

Here are some other factors researchers believe may affect the forging of a bond (and remember, it's a two-way street):

• The mother's ability to interpret the baby's signals. Most new mothers soon learn to tell the difference between a baby's cry when he's hungry and his cry when he's wet or otherwise uncomfortable. This sensitivity helps a baby learn to be both dependent on his mother and confident that she'll meet his needs.

• The mother's personality. The warmer she is, the easier it will be for her and the baby to bond; the more anxious and fearful, the more difficult.

• How the mother was raised. How did your mother respond to *you*? This can shape your own style of relating to your baby.

• How the mother feeds the baby. Many researchers believe that breastfeeding is a big aid in the bonding process,
partly because of the physical closeness it engenders and
partly because it makes the baby totally dependent on only
the mother for sustenance. Some researchers have even
found evidence that prolactin, the hormone responsible for
milk secretion, may also actually trigger some types of
maternal behavior.

Mary Ainsworth, a psychologist at Johns Hopkins University, told *Parents* magazine that she believes that the
manner in which a mother feeds her child—and not necessarily the vehicle, be it breast or bottle—is an indicator of
the quality of the attachment the mother has to her child.
Ainsworth said she's observed that a mother who responds
quickly to her baby's cries of hunger and who then at-
tempts to make the feeding pleasant for the infant seems
more responsive to that infant in most other situations as
well, in comparison to the mother who doesn't respond as
readily to her baby's hunger.

Okay, so what if you're sitting there and your baby is six
weeks old and you still don't feel that the two of you are
particularly close? Try not to worry. It will happen in time.
Apparently, many a new mother cannot really relate to her
baby until the baby recognizes and responds to her as an
individual. One mother I interviewed provided a perfect
example of this: "In the first few months of my baby's life,"
she said, "I was secretly very resentful that she didn't care
who fed her and that my husband and I could go away for
a weekend and leave her with my mother and she didn't
even seem to notice the difference. We'd come home and
my mother would say, 'Oh, she smiled so much and slept
and ate like a little angel' and it was a knife in my heart.
Then, when she was about six or seven months old, she

suddenly began to cry whenever I'd leave the room, even if it was just to duck into the pantry for half a second. Publicly, I pretended to be exasperated by this behavior, but inside I was thrilled. It was then that I first felt those fierce, chest-swelling feelings like *I'll always, always, always be here for you, Babe.*"

The End of Maternity Leave

For many women, the worst emotional upheaval during the first year postpartum occurs when it's time to go back to work and entrust the baby's care to someone else. It's a situation that most new mothers face these days: according to the 1990 U.S. Census, 53.1 percent of working women return to their jobs before the baby's first birthday; among women with college degrees that figure is 68 percent.

Many women are surprised at how having a baby changes their perspective about work. "I always believed that nothing could be more fulfilling and exciting than working in advertising," one told me. "Never in my wildest dreams had I imagined myself wanting to be a stay-at-home mom." And yet, when this woman went back to work she lasted all of three hours. She went home and stayed home for five years.

Most mothers who return to work, even those who want to, experience a profound sense of loss. "My feelings were on a par with the grief I felt when my beloved grandmother died," a woman told me. "I was literally mourning the end of a very special time in my life and my daughter's. Every three hours, my breasts would ache as if in accusation: 'You should be home with her.' I'd hole up in a stall in the women's restroom, pump them dry, and silently weep that I was in that cold, ugly place instead of rocking and singing to my daughter as she nursed in the sunny corner of her bedroom."

Besides loss, other feelings you may grapple with when you return to work are resentment (that your husband doesn't make enough money to allow you to stay home, for example) and anxiety (perhaps that your baby is being neglected or mistreated by her new caregiver). Some mothers wrestle with guilt that they *like* being out of the house and back at work. Kathie Lee Gifford, cohost of "Live with Regis and Kathie Lee," experienced several of these emotions when she returned to work five weeks after her first child, Cody, was born. "If I gave up my career I would hate to think that someday I might blame Cody and say 'You kept my dreams from coming true,'" she wrote in her 1992 autobiography *I Can't Believe I Said That!* (Pocket Books). "It's a tough balance to strike between regretting what I miss at home if I work and resenting what's at home if I don't."

After returning to the job, most mothers go through a transitional period when they find it difficult to concentrate on work. A New York book editor I know described her inability to think about anything but her baby in her first weeks back to a journalist who was writing an article on this very subject. My editor friend was horrified when she discovered that, thanks to a misunderstanding with the journalist, she was quoted and fully identified—by first and last name—in the lead paragraph of the story, which was published in a major women's magazine. "Suddenly, everyone in the company was aware of the fact that they'd been paying me to just sit there and think about my daughter," the editor said with a wry laugh. "Luckily, no one called me on it."

All of these feelings can and usually do bring on a bout

of depression, but mothers who have been there say it lifts a little with each passing day. Some of their advice:

If possible, ease back into the job gradually. If you have any option for going back less than full time, take it for a few months.

Find the highest-quality, most trustworthy childcare you can afford. "This won't make you feel any less sad, but at least you won't be worried sick on top of everything else," a mother told me.

On this same subject, many women fear that the baby will begin to prefer the caregiver. But according to Jay Belsky, Ph.D., a professor of human development at Penn State who's done numerous studies on the effects of childcare on children, "There is no evidence that a baby will become more attached to the caregiver than to the mother. The few studies that have been done in this area clearly indicate that babies have preferences for their mothers."

Still, according to San Francisco psychologist Lin Yeiser, there *is* a slight possibility that a child will grow to prefer the caregiver. "You can prevent this from happening by trying not to go back to work before your child can recognize you consistently, at about four months," said Yeiser, author of *Nannies, Au Pairs, Mother's Helpers—Caregivers: The Complete Guide to Home Child Care.* "It's even better if you can wait until his attachment to you is fully formed at six months. If waiting isn't possible, spend as much off-work time with him as possible, attending to his needs and building your relationship."

Keep telling yourself that your working is in your child's best interests. If you have to return to work for financial reasons, try to keep in mind that your working allows you to feed, clothe, and shelter your child properly and will perhaps even provide her with a good head start in her adult life in the form of financial help with a college education.

If you're returning to work for other than financial reasons, remind yourself of these words from eminent pediatrician T. Berry Brazelton: "There are benefits for every member of the family when a woman feels fulfilled," he said in *Working and Caring* (Addison-Wesley). "Research clearly demonstrates that, if a woman is successful and happy at work, she is more likely to be successful at home, and as a mother." In her book *Mother Care/Other Care* (Basic Books), University of Virginia psychologist Sandra Scarr mentions that several studies show that the most frustrated and depressed mothers are those who are non-employed who wish they could get out of the house to a workplace. Then she says, "Depressed mothers have depressing effects on their children. Children of depressed mothers avoid them and shun attention from other adults." She also cites a study that found that such children seem to develop an avoidance of emotional involvements with others.

Let's drag Kathie Lee Gifford back into this discussion. She said she had a little help from her mother in getting over her guilt about wanting to return to work after her son Cody was born. As Gifford told *Ladies' Home Journal*: "She said, 'Honey, even though I was always home [when you were growing up], if you think you had my undivided attention, you're crazy. I was cooking, I was cleaning, I was on the phone, and I had two other children. As long as Cody is a happy and well-adjusted little boy, you're doing it right.' It was such a gift from her to say that."

Possessed!

One very common but almost never discussed emotional side effect of childbirth in the first year (or more) is that you can become like a person possessed; you can be so totally absorbed in motherhood and your baby that the rest of the world seems to fade away completely.

A woman whose baby was born shortly before the Persian Gulf War started in January 1991 told me she was "barely aware there was a war going on, except for the fact that my sports junkie husband was, for once, constantly tuned to CNN instead of ESPN. The bombing raids on Israel, the press conferences with the generals—it was all just meaningless, murmuring background noise to me. About a year after my daughter was born, I read old *Time* magazines about that war with rapt fascination, sort of like a Rip Van Winkle who was finally coming back to life after a long sleep and was eager to find out everything he'd missed."

As writer Janet Spencer King once put it in *Parents* magazine, "Just as very young infants don't realize the first few months that they are not a part of Mother, in an emotional sense, it's not much different for their moms." She goes on to quote the late British psychoanalyst D. W. Winnicott as describing this total absorption in the new mother as a "normal illness" and one whose intensity is difficult for the woman to recall once she has "recovered" from it.

I myself may not remember the intensity of the experience, but I do remember certain bizarre and inconsiderate actions I took while I was a person possessed, including one that still fills me with guilt. When Madeline was about three months old, one of my best friends called, worried sick, because she'd found a lump in her breast a week earlier and it hadn't disappeared after her period. I remember distractedly telling her not to worry about it, that it was probably just an infection in a milk duct. Then I had to hang up because the baby was crying. Well, a woman who has not given birth and who is not breastfeeding cannot have an infection in a milk duct, so that was an idiotic response—especially from someone who had for years been writing articles about women's special health concerns. But I was so caught up in my own breastfeeding that the error of my response just didn't occur to me. Nor did I remember to follow up with this worried friend. It was another year before I learned that she went on to have three separate mammograms and that after one of those, her doctor said "I'm afraid this lump looks terribly suspicious. But let's just wait and see." Fortunately, it turned out to be benign, but that was yet another thing I didn't know—and failed to inquire about—at the time. While this friend good-naturedly continued to call me and meet me for lunch during that first postpartum year, she instinctively kept the conversation light, as if she knew I wouldn't be much good at anything heavy that didn't concern motherhood in general and my baby in particular. If one good thing came out of all this, it's that the patience and understanding she demonstrated eventually made me appreciate my friend and our friendship more than ever.

I was not so lucky with another friend, someone with whom I'd been through cross-country moves, corporate reorganizations, and love life trials and triumphs for ten years. I lost her within a year of Madeline's birth. I remember her making resentful noises whenever I'd change the subject and start talking about the baby or, worse, would insist on bringing Madeline along on shopping or lunch jaunts. I, in turn, made resentful noises about her resentful noises to another friend, the mother of a two-year-old. This fellow mother said, "She's probably just jealous that you have a baby and she doesn't."

It was years before it hit me that it was far more likely that what drove her away was not jealousy but mind-numbing, eye-glazing, hair-tearing *boredom*. Discourses on Pampers versus Huggies, whether a 2T and 24 months are really the same size, and when to initiate potty training are utterly and crashingly uninteresting to most women who have never had babies, and even to a lot of women who have. When my friend Stephanie's second child was about nine months old, she joined a playgroup of other mothers with nine-month-old babies, but all of the other women were first-time mothers. Stephanie lasted only two play dates. "All they could talk about were their babies!" she reported. "I felt like standing up and shouting 'Get a life!'"

When *do* you get a life? When do you snap out of it and join the human race again? Well, mentally, you'll never really go back to the way you were prebaby; motherhood will forever change the way you see the world (read more about this in Chapter 9). But eventually, the baby will stop being your entire world. Postpartum researcher and Washington, D.C., therapist Elizabeth Zinner told *Parents* that by nine months, most babies become interested in the world beyond their mothers and that "as babies begin to turn outward, the mothers start to involve themselves in their own lives, too."

Or, as my friend Glenda put it, "At your child's first birthday, your friends will also secretly be celebrating the fact that you are no longer a pod person."

Another friend of mine feels that the very nature of friendship has to change after one friend has a baby and that some "nonmom" friends find it difficult to adjust. "I had one friend who expected me to be the same after giving birth," she said. "She acted shocked and amazed when I said something funny to her about six months after my daughter was born. She said, 'You have your sense of humor back!' I thought that was unnecessarily harsh. It's hard to be funny when you're working plus nursing six times a day."

My friend added that she attributed this attitude in friends without children not to jealousy but to a total lack of comprehension of the totality of change a baby wreaks on one's life. "It's almost impossible to be as good or thoughtful a friend postbaby, because someone's *life* now depends on you. Your time is no longer your own, your worries are more mundane (money, your marriage, being a good parent). It's hard to be interesting to others when your concerns are so personal. Though you are more selfish prebaby, you *seem* less so!"

CHAPTER EIGHT

THE ZEN OF MOTHERHOOD
Doing 100 Different Things at Once

Life in the United States is rush-rush for everybody these days. But adding the responsibility for the well-being and entertainment of another human being to everything else an adult woman must do puts motherhood in a class by itself. Perhaps "doing 100 different things at once" is an exaggeration. But I assure you that for at least the first few years of your child's life you will rarely if ever enjoy the luxury of doing just one thing at a time.

You will read the paper while you feed your baby her cereal. You will help your child practice her song for the Christmas pageant while you cook dinner. You will remove the cellophane from a box of juice and insert the straw while driving and then mop up the juice that was squirted all over the car while you're merging onto the freeway. You will bake cookies for the preschool, write thank-you notes for your child's birthday presents, and talk to your mother on the phone while you watch TV. And that's just your *physical* activity. All the while, you'll also be trying to keep in mind that your child needs a third dose of "the pink stuff" (antibiotic) before she goes to bed, that you need to schedule that follow-up on her ear infection with the pediatrician within the next two days, that you must RSVP to a friend's wedding by the fourteenth, and that you won't be able to mail out all those thank-you notes you're writing unless you stop at the post office in the morning.

I love the way Ann Pleshette Murphy, editor-in-chief of *Parents* magazine, once described a mother's brain. It seems a friend she had not seen for a while asked her what she'd been up to, and Murphy tried to describe her multiple roles as wife, mother, editor, writer, manager, volunteer, and school board member. The friend said, "You must have a very full head."

Wrote Murphy in *Parents*: "I immediately conjured up the image of one of those old steamer trunks lined with dozens of little drawers and compartments and I had to admit that every single compartment was jammed. In one, there was a list of groceries I needed to pick up on my way home. In another was a growing pile of pink phone-message slips. And then there were the gifts to send, articles to read, library books to return, doctors' appointments to make, letters to write—not to mention the stuff that couldn't be compartmentalized, such as spontaneous hugs from my kids and a quiet conversation with my husband."

Said a friend: "Nobody ever tells you that *every* day of motherhood will be the equivalent of the most stressful, hair-tearing, tired-to-the-bone, but only *occasional* day in your old life. Not only must your body perform on double time, so must your mind. You have to learn to live with your mind on fast-forward: 'What six completely unrelated tasks must I accomplish in the next two hours?'"

That fast-forward mode has its consequences. For some moms, it's a sort of constant mental fuzziness, the vague feeling that brain power isn't what it once was. For me, a woman who once prided herself on her excellent memory, it's absentmindedness. Before I had Madeline, I never once forgot to write a check down in my register; nowadays, at least once a month I'm on the phone to the bank asking, "Did check number 326 clear yet, and if so for what amount?" Many mothers have described incidents to me of walking into another room or even driving across the city and completely forgetting what motivated the trip in the first place! I remember laughing with almost hysterical relief and empathy when the fellow mother of an eighteen-month-old quaveringly confessed that she feared she was in the early stages of Alzheimer's disease. Likewise, I absolutely howled with delight when I read this passage in Anne Lamott's *Operating Instructions: A Journal of My Son's First Year* (Pantheon): "It's been 26 years since John Kennedy was killed. I was in fifth grade. I had a chopped olive sandwich for lunch and two Hostess cupcakes. I can remember all that exactly, and yet a few days ago I got into the shower in my underpants."

Motherhood stress can manifest itself in crabbiness, too. "Do you ever have days where instead of feeling like your kid's mom you feel like a really mean big sister?" is the way my friend Rachel once put it to me.

Another mom told me, "My husband and I flash past each other in the hall like ships in the night—make that *jet boats* in the night. When we do have a minute together, we snipe at each other over the stupidest little things. And every night as we collapse into bed, we have this sort of unofficial contest: who has more of a right to feel completely and totally exhausted? I'll say, 'I did this and this and this today' and he'll say, 'Oh, yeah? Well, I did this and this and this.' It's a parenthood version of 'My dog's bigger than your dog.'"

Several moms told me that the stress of motherhood leaves them susceptible to frequent bouts of feeling inadequate. "Because of lack of time, I can never give anything 100 percent anymore, and as a result I feel like I do nothing really well these days," said Maria, a writer friend. "Like I'll mail out a manuscript hating the fact that there's a typo on page 7 but having no time to fix it. Or, as a gift, I'll buy someone a book that's simply on the bestseller list and feel guilty about not being able to search for a book that would really interest that particular person. Or instead of rolling out dough and cutting out pumpkin-shaped cookies for the preschool Halloween party, I'll have to throw together the kind you can just drop from a spoon onto the cookie sheet, and then I'll plunk a pumpkin candy in the middle of each. The result looks really dumb, and I know all the other moms think so, too."

Deborah Shaw Lewis, a Rome, Georgia, stay-at-home mother of five, wrote an entire book on this subject. In *Motherhood Stress* (Word Publishing) she identifies several key features that make this kind of stress unique. I'll list a few of these, along with my own comments and examples.

Unpredictability. For example, you have your day carefully planned down to the last minute, and all of a sudden your toddler—smiling and babbling cheerfully just seconds earlier—throws up all over your minivan.

Lack of control. Researchers have determined that the people who have the least amount of control in their jobs are the most stressed. Ever see a mother trying to deal with a toddler who is throwing a tantrum in the supermarket?

There's never enough time. Syndicated columnist Ellen Goodman once wrote that what most mothers would really, truly love for Mother's Day is *time*. "A gift box of an extra hour would be nice," she said, "or a day off, placed at the edge of the bed tray, next to the burnt pancakes and the handmade card."

Lack of time made Bree Walker—a familiar face if you watch TV news in New York City, Los Angeles, or San Diego—commit an almost unpardonable sin for a female news anchor: she cut off her long hair without asking the station's permission. Walker had wrestled with the decision for almost a year before that, but it had finally come down to a simple choice: her kids or her hair. "You're standing there doing your hair and your baby is crying," she told the *Los Angeles Times*. "The last thing I need is guilt over my damn long hair. I needed more time for my kids. And I bought 45 minutes a day in my life by cutting off my hair."

Power overload. The very idea that you're responsible for someone else's physical, emotional, social, and spiritual health can be overwhelming.

Poor job training. As the actress Cher, mother of Chastity and Elijah Blue, once put it in *New Woman* magazine, "That line in 'Mermaids'—'You guys didn't come with instructions'—that's my line. It is hard when you're trying to do the best you can; [being a mother is] one of the many things you need to learn but no one teaches you in school." There is no "Introduction to Colic," no "Dealing with Finicky Eaters 101."

Unrealistic expectations. We want to be "perfect" mothers. We want to be like Carol Brady (of "The Brady Bunch"). And when we're not—when we shout "Because

I'm the mother, that's why!" or we make drop cookies or buy Chips Ahoy instead of baking the cookie-cutter kind— we feel guilty and/or inadequate, and/or we drive ourselves even harder. What we forget is that Carol Brady had a full-time live-in (remember Alice?). At least our daughters are growing up with more realistic "role models," like Marge Simpson and Roseanne.

Inadequate feedback. It's frustrating to not know how well you're doing the job. There's no report card like you had in school or annual performance review like you have on the job. It may seem as if the only feedback you get is critical: "If you keep picking her up whenever she cries, you'll spoil her!"

Low status. It's also frustrating to be unappreciated. If you want a concrete example of just how low-status taking care of children is, here's one: According to the U.S. Department of Labor, Bureau of Labor Statistics, the median annual salary for a full-time childcare provider in the United States is $10,150.

On the home front, consider the couples I know in which the husband goes off to a job and the wife stays home with the kids. In probably 75 percent of the cases, after each has put in a full eight hours of hard work, the husband comes home and plops down on the couch to watch or read the news or simply disappears into some far corner of the house for thirty or forty minutes while the wife just keeps right on working—often for three to five more hours. What is the implication here? That *his* work is clearly the more important, the more deserving of a "break," because he is *paid* for it.

To Complicate Matters

What could possibly increase motherhood stress even more? Two things: a job outside the home and/or having more than one child. And both of these factors are the reality for most mothers.

I recently read a quote from a male sociologist to the effect that "what makes life so stressful these days is that you have two people, husband and wife, trying to do three jobs—the paycheck job of each plus managing the household." Well, I beg to differ. If recent surveys are any indication, just *one* of those persons is doing two jobs. According to recent surveys conducted by *Redbook* and *Working Mother* magazines:

- 94 percent of wives buy all of the kids' clothes

- 93 percent make the kids' doctors appointments

- 92 percent do the laundry

- 82 percent clean the house

- 79 percent prepare all the meals

- 71 percent do all the dishes

Some more telling statistics: only about 10 percent of couples share household jobs equally, according to the Wellesley College Center for Research on Women. And women are not very happy about the situation. A 1990 Roper poll showed that 52 percent of female respondents resent their husbands for not doing more housework and seven out of ten believe that if they did get more help, it would be a heckuva lot easier to juggle work, marriage, and children. And get this: not only do most men do a minimal amount of work around the house, they evidently *generate* more work for their wives. How else can you explain the study that found that single mothers spend less time on chores (sixteen hours a week) than their married counterparts (twenty hours a week)? Finally, there's this eye-opener: husbands do the same amount of housework whether their wives work or not, according to two separate university studies.

What all this means is that after a mother puts in her eight hours at work, she comes home to what sociologist Alice Hochschild calls "the second shift": childcare, housework, and cooking. Sandra Scarr, the University of Virginia psychology professor who wrote *Mother Care/Other Care*, has said that "many working mothers' daily lives make sweatshop labor look like a vacation."

Now throw an extra kid or two into the equation. Said one mom: "You know how people say having two kids doesn't just double your work load, it quadruples it? Once I had my own second child, I realized why that's true. Let me give you just one example: Until our second child was born, we just picked up our older child's toys once a day, usually right before bedtime. But after the baby was born we had to keep picking up the older one's toys constantly because we were afraid the baby would get ahold of something he could choke on."

Added my friend Rachel, "Having two is as different from having one as having one is from having none. You spend an awful lot of time trying to help your first adjust to the second and a lot of time making sure the second isn't cheated out of all the nurturing you gave the first. And since you *can't* give the second as much as you gave the first, you feel guilty."

"You know how much control over your life you relinquished with the first?" another friend asked me. "You relinquish that much more again with the second. For example, before I had kids I was never more than a minute or two late to anything if I was late at all. After my first child, being five minutes late became standard. Since my second child, no matter how organized I try to be, that five minutes has permanently increased to ten. For most of the first year of my second child's life, I felt like I was in this dark tunnel, relinquishing more control every day."

This all sounds very daunting and dismal. The good news is, however, that once your second child reaches the age of nine months or a year, things get a lot easier, according to most moms of more than one. Said my "dark tunnel" friend: "Suddenly, you don't have to sterilize everything anymore, or to haul fifty pounds of diapers and other gear whenever you leave the house. You no longer have to wash the baby's clothes separately, and he's walking and playing with your first so that they're entertaining each other. Best of all, he's sleeping for seven or eight hours at a stretch at night."

"I've developed amnesia for how crazy I felt the first year of John's life," said Rachel about her second, who was fourteen months old when she said this. "That sense of chaos and exhaustion is just gone. Know how I knew it was over? I started having yearnings for a *third* child."

Preventing Stress from Becoming Distress

There are other things you can do, however, to decrease motherhood stress besides just waiting for your child to get older. These are not just things you can do but things that you *should* do, because stress not only makes you more susceptible to nuisances such as headaches and the common cold (75 to 90 percent of all physician visits are made because of stress-related ailments), it's also linked to big-

time problems such as ulcers, cancer, heart disease, and
high blood pressure.

Okay, but let's say you're not a raving, hysterical harri-
dan who spends most of her waking hours shrieking at the
kids, husband, preschool teacher, and women in cleaning
product commercials on TV. How then do you tell whether
you're stressed, or just plain busy? Shirley Dunn, a Lenox,
Massachusetts–based nurse who is a consultant to companies on stress management, told *Parents* magazine that the
symptoms of stress fall into four categories: physical, emotional, psychological, and behavioral. Common physical
symptoms include acne, fatigue, and dizziness. Emotional
symptoms might be anxiety, depression, fear, impatience, a
sense of isolation, or a feeling that no one understands you.
Psychological symptoms, said Dunn, might include indecision, insecurity, self-rejecting thoughts, and diminished
creativity. Finally, behavioral signs of too much stress can
be overeating, abusing alcohol or drugs, irritability, and/or
procrastination.

Any one or a combination of these may be a warning
that you need to make some changes in your life. In the
rest of this chapter, let's look at several ideas:

Dealing with Everyday Annoyances

Avoid predictably stressful situations. Do your shopping
and banking during off-hours, if possible, when lines are
shorter. Get an answering machine to screen your calls at
home, and make it a rule that no one can answer the phone
during dinner. Buy extra birthday gifts and a box of all-
occasion cards so that you won't have to rush out at the
last minute when your child suddenly reminds you, "Today
is Mikey's birthday party." By the same token, stock up on

absolute essentials such as tampons and toilet paper. Make duplicates of all of your keys and always carry spare change in your car.

Talk to yourself. If you can't avoid a stressful situation, try to calmly put your negative feelings into words, such as "I'm upset because I'm stuck in traffic and I have a hundred things to do tonight." Then try to come up with at least ten ways to make the situation more tolerable, such as (1) "I could get off the freeway and take Route 1," (2) "I could buy cookies for Jenny's class instead of baking them," and so on. You probably have more options than you originally thought.

Use humor. A Long Island company called Stresscare that conducts stress management seminars has come up with a way to prompt a laugh and diffuse a stressful situation. With their "blow up" method, you mentally blow a stressful situation all out of proportion until it's ludicrous. For example, if you feel your hackles rising because you've already been waiting in a bank line ten minutes, tell yourself, "I'll probably be in this line until I'm old and they have to wheel me outside in a wheelchair, where I'll answer reporters' questions about how it feels to be going into the *Guinness Book of Records* as The Person Who Stood in Line the Longest. And I'll say 'Pretty good, especially since by the time I got up to the teller I was so old the teller offered me an interest-free senior citizens checking account!'"

Recast delays as opportunities. Use waiting room and stand-in-line time for reading your favorite magazine or writing a letter to a friend.

Don't waste stress on people and situations over which you have no control. According to Jerome Murray, a clinical psychologist in Santa Rosa, California, everybody is born with a genetically determined amount of stress-coping energy. As this energy is depleted, he says, the physiological toll that depletion takes is that you age, and when it's gone you die. "The next time you impotently rage at the 'idiot' going 40 in the fast lane," said Murray in *USA Today* magazine, "ask yourself 'Is it really worth it? It could cost you seconds of your life. Do you really want to waste your finite stress-coping energy on someone you don't even know?'"

Making Your Life Easier

Make lists—but set priorities. Many moms swear by making a daily list of what needs to be done. But such a list can seem overwhelming if it gets too long. That's why you should organize the list: make the first task the one that has the highest penalty should you be late in doing it; the second item has the next-worst penalty, and so on. For example, the penalty if you don't "Call Mom to wish her a happy birthday" is probably greater than the twenty-five cents you'll have to pay if you fail to "Return the library book due today."

Establish routines. Routines are important, especially for the two prime stress times of the day: early morning and bedtime. For example, you always head the kids up to bed at 7:45, you supervise as they brush their teeth, you read them one story, then they have ten minutes to look at books on their own before it's lights out at 8:30.

You have to adopt routines and keep things on a schedule if you ever want to carve out regular free time for yourself. In addition, if kids know what to expect, you cut down on wheedling, whining, and dawdling—all stress producers. One additional benefit: psychologists say routines give children a sense of security, stability, and trust.

Have regular family meetings. Meet every Tuesday night, for example. Regular family meetings should serve a dual purpose. They should cover the operation of "The Firm" (as Queen Elizabeth refers to her family) to deal with such practical matters as where to take this year's vacation and how to cut family food costs. The more efficiently the household runs, the less stress for you. The regular family meeting is also the time to discuss any tensions or conflicts that have arisen, so that they don't become chronic sources of resentment and stress. Even three- and four-year-olds may have concerns and they should be allowed to express them.

Be specific about assigning chores. Don't just say "Jason, I want you to start helping me at dinnertime." Be specific. Say "I want you to start clearing the table and loading the dinner dishes into the dishwasher." As family therapist David C. Treadway put it in the *Harvard Family Health Letter*, "If tasks are not assigned, they are constantly open for negotiation, which can send the stress level skyrocketing."

Get your husband to help more. When you are enlisting your husband's help, once again be specific. Don't just say "I want more help from you." Make it "Since I'm the one who always cooks dinner, I'd like you to be the one who always cleans up afterward."

If you do get him to help, don't criticize his methods. Criticism will give him an excuse to stop doing the chore, as in "You don't like the way I do it, so it's probably easier if you just do it yourself." On one particularly frantic morning when Madeline was three, Steve offered to get her dressed for preschool, which had always been my domain. While Steve has faultless taste in his own clothes, he somehow saw nothing wrong with pairing an orange and red plaid shirt with a pair of pink corduroy overalls that were so short you could see the tops of her socks (I'd kept them around to be used as "paint" clothes). Since Madeline didn't complain (she didn't adopt her own rigid dress code till about 4½), I kept my mouth shut. I had to bite my lip to keep from laughing when her teacher took one look at her and whispered to me, "Good for you! Letting children make their own decisions about what to wear, no matter how terrible their choices, is a good way to teach independence."

Some moms swear by the I-can-stand-it-longer-than-you-can method, in which you simply stop doing a chore, such as the laundry, until your husband—desperate for clean socks—breaks down and does it himself. ("This didn't work for me," one mother reported. "When my husband found out he had no more clean underwear, he just went out and bought new ones!")

And then there are the more creative ways of getting your husband (and your kids, if they're old enough) to help. Marilyn Kentz, one-half of the stand-up comedy duo known as "The Mommies," once served an entire dinner (lamb chops and all) directly on the table because the other members of the family repeatedly failed to set the table. "They never forgot after that," she told *People*.

Several mothers told me they got dad to help with childcare by regularly leaving him alone with the baby from the very start. This quickly makes him feel confident about his ability to take care of the child and also establishes a bond between them, a bond he will want to keep up by continuing to participate in the child's care and entertainment over the years.

What if your husband simply refuses to help with child-care or housework? Then you must simply insist that the two of you rework the family budget in order to find the money to hire the help you need.

Lower your standards. You will not be arrested if you fail to include each of the four food groups in every meal, nor will your child grow up to be two inches shorter than she could have been. If you're feeling overwhelmed at dinner-time and didn't make it to the store, serve corn flakes. Or have a pizza delivered. Take some of the pressure off yourself by not expecting perfection.

Eliminate "have-to-do's." Eliminating some of the things you "have to" do goes hand in hand with lowering your standards. Make a list of all the regular chores you do, noting how often you do them. Now try to determine if you can do them less frequently. Do you have to empty all the wastebaskets every week, particularly since they're never more than half-full? Will you (or anybody else) notice the difference if you stop washing the sheets every Saturday and go to twice a month?

Learn to say no. You can say no without saying "No!" What I've found works is to just say in a harried, semihys-terical, somewhat breathless voice, "Look, I wish I could help but I can't. I'm simply overwhelmed." I leave what I'm overwhelmed by to the caller's imagination.

You really don't owe anyone an explanation for saying no to a request for your time, especially if you know darn well that saying yes is going to make your life even crazier.

Experts advise asking yourself a handful of questions before saying yes to a request for your time: Do I *have* to do this? Will I enjoy doing this? Is this project important to me? Do I have the energy and time for it? If your answer to any one of these is no, then you should seriously consider making that your final answer.

If you can't bring yourself to say an outright no, always respond to a request with something like "I'll have to check my schedule and get back to you." Not only will this protect you from saying yes because you were caught off guard, it gives you the opportunity to come up with an excuse for not accepting the person's request if you really don't want to. For example, you can then call the person back and say, "I'm sorry, but I checked my schedule and I'm busy that day" (because you're busy *every* day!).

Seize control wherever you can. Many facets of motherhood can't be controlled (such as just when your child will come down with chicken pox). But you can retain some sense of control over your life by instilling order wherever you can. Clean out your closet or Rolodex. Organize your spice cabinet. Keep the top of your desk free of clutter. Where to find the time? One idea: turn the task into a game you can play with your child. Example: "Let's pile all the sweaters in this corner, all the pants on the bed, all the dresses in this box. . . . "

Turning the Heat Down

Do something fun at least once a week. Lyle Miller, Ph.D., Alma Dell Smith, Ph.D., and Larry Rothman, Ed.D., who wrote the book *The Stress Solution* (Pocket Books/Simon & Schuster) say their research indicates that "people who do something enjoyable at least once a week experience less stress from the demands and pressures of family, feel better about themselves, have less marital turmoil, and have fewer symptoms of stress than those who report they never have fun."

Don't try to make every minute with your child meaningful. Sirgay Sanger, M.D., a psychiatrist and coauthor of the book *The Woman Who Works, The Parent Who Cares* (Harper & Row), has said that it's really helpful for stressed-out parents to remember that a parent's job is to love her child, not educate him. "The notion that time with our child should be productive is very stressful," he said in *Parents* magazine. "You don't need to 'accomplish' anything when you're with your children." Just hanging out together is enough.

Don't put off tough decisions. As I write this, two of my friends, fellow mothers of five-year-olds, are agonizing over whether they should send their children to kindergarten this fall or wait another year. Experts say that indecision itself creates stress and that not making a decision is frequently more stressful than making a "wrong" choice. So, don't put off making hard decisions.

Give yourself a pep talk. A lot of stress is self-inflicted, thanks to the negative and often self-deprecating comments we make when we're talking to ourselves, such as "I just cannot cope with all this" or "My family doesn't appreciate all I do." You can wrest yourself out of this state by drowning out such thoughts with positive ones: "I can, too!" or "I've really accomplished a lot today."

England's "Fergie" apparently used this technique during the most stressful and scandalous periods that she was in the public spotlight. According to the book *Fergie Con-*

fidential, she would look in the mirror every morning and ask herself "Who loves you, baby?" She would respond with the names of her family. Then she would ask herself two more questions: "What are you most proud of?" and "What are you glad about today?" Said Fergie, "By the time I have answered, I feel much happier. It sets me up for the day."

Rely on the three P's: pets, people, and parks. James Lynch, a researcher at the University of Maryland, has found that just petting your dog or cat is a natural stress reliever. It slows your heart rate and lowers your blood pressure.

Having at least one close, trusted friend to confide in is also important. According to one study, women who are under severe stress and don't have somebody to confide in are twice as likely to be depressed as women who are equally stressed but who do have a confidante.

If you have no friend available but find yourself at the end of your rope in dealing with your child on a particularly exasperating day, seek the sympathy and fellowship of other parents at your local park. As writer Joyce Maynard once put it, this is "why playgrounds—or any other place that encourages young children and parents to gather—are as important for grownups as they are for kids." And the park can serve another useful purpose when you're battling stress. Read on.

Take a walk. Walk in the park, or just around your neighborhood. A brisk fifteen-minute walk has been found to be more calming than the tranquilizer meprobamate (Equinil). And regular walking, actually regular exercise of any sort, helps the body adapt more readily to stress. A fit body pumps out lesser amounts of the "fight or flight" hormones that produce stress symptoms such as the jitters and sweating.

Stop worrying. If you find yourself frequently fretting about what-if scenarios, here's a simple exercise suggested by *Working Woman* magazine: Rank the events that are bothering you in order of severity and assess their probability of happening. Wait a month; then review the list as a reality check. This exercise should help you become adept at identifying and dismissing these worries for what they are—imaginary.

Don't bottle up your emotions. According to the authors of *The Stress Solution*, repressing anger, anxiety, or depression decreases your resistance to stress. Get things off your chest.

My husband, Steve, has a very logical and scientific mind, and I have found it a great relief to have him calmly analyze and dissect my frequent anxieties about Madeline. For example, I'll tell him "I'm worried sick that the Smiths aren't watching Madeline and that she'll wander out to their backyard, fall into the pool, and drown." And he'll say, "That's not going to happen because, one, they have a childproof lock on that back door and, two, Madeline wouldn't go out there anyway because she's afraid of their dog; and three . . . ," and so on.

Sit down and watch "Mister Rogers' Neighborhood." I know it's popular to make fun of Mister Rogers, but I'm not being facetious here. I've witnessed three- and four-year-old hellions turn angelic and docile when this PBS program comes on, thanks to Fred Rogers' consistently gentle and unhurried voice and manner. It works for moms, too; at least it does for this mom. I don't even have to really listen to what he's saying. I can read the paper or whatever, and just the cadence of his voice in the background calms me down.

Pay your childcare provider. If you're not paying your childcare provider, consider switching to paid care. One of the most surprising findings of a 1990 *Redbook* survey on women and stress was that, among women who work and use childcare, those who use an *unpaid* relative or friend are the most stressed. Why? Stress researcher Deborah Belle of Boston University speculated for *Redbook* that women who don't pay for childcare may feel they don't have a right to complain about facets of that care that they don't like (remember, bottled-up emotions produce stress), and criticizing a relative or a friend who means well is difficult to do even when those services are paid for.

So it just may be worth your while, if not your sanity, to switch from your sister to a local professional or high-quality day-care center.

Take a music break. Scientists believe that playing calm music in the operating room reduces the amount of anesthesia patients need, because it has a tranquilizing effect. Try it at home whenever you have a few spare minutes to just sit, relax, and listen. You don't have to settle for "elevator music," but opt for something that's slow, nonvocal, and quiet for best results. "The all-time favorite in our house, even among the teens," one mom told me, "is Pachelbel's 'Canon in D Major.' Canons are mesmerizing."

Try a relaxation exercise. There are three that work particularly well:

• Visual imagery. Close your eyes and picture yourself back in the most relaxing place you've ever been in your

life. Conjure up and enjoy every vivid detail you recall—
the feel of the sun on your back, the sound of the waves
lapping up on the shore, and so on. Stay there for at least
five minutes.

• Progressive muscle relaxation. This one is based on the
principle that a muscle will relax automatically after it is
tightened forcefully. Lie down and concentrate on tightening your forehead for five seconds, then relax it. Progress
down your body, one part at a time: tighten and relax your
jaw, your neck, your shoulders, all the way to your toes. Try
to devote at least fifteen minutes to this exercise.

• The Relaxation Response. Herbert Benson, a Harvard
researcher, devised this exercise because he's found that
when people meditate, a feeling of tranquility washes over
them—and muscle tension, heart rate, brain-wave activity,
and blood pressure all decrease. Find a quiet part of the
house where you can be alone for at least ten minutes and
preferably twenty. If your husband isn't available to watch
your child, wait for naptime or "Sesame Street." Close your
eyes and repeat silently (or whisper) a meaningless word or
phrase (you may wish to use the universal mantra "om")
over and over again. Try to concentrate only on that sound;
if an intrusive thought drifts in, simply say to yourself,
"Oh, well," let it drift out, and return to repeating and
focusing on the mantra.

Incidentally, you can also use the Relaxation Response to
help you fall asleep at night. In one study, seven out of ten
people who were suffering severe insomnia were able to
achieve normal sleep patterns by using this exercise.

• Pop bubbles. This is no joke: A recent study at Western
New England College in Springfield, Massachusetts, found
that students were less tense and more calm and energized

after popping sheets of bubble wrap, the plastic packing material with sealed-air capsules that we all know and love. I was tickled to hear about this since Madeline, Steve, and I have long been addicted to popping bubble wrap, fighting over these sheets like puppies when the mail arrives. Study participants preferred popping the larger bubbles over the smaller variety—the pop is more satisfying. Kathleen Dillon, Ph.D., the professor of psychology who directed the study, told *Glamour* that popping the plastic bubbles is in the same league as knitting, finger tapping, and fiddling with worry beads—all activities that dispel muscle tension and pent-up nervous energy. She added that bubble popping has advantages over more conventional de-stressing techniques, such as meditation, because no instruction or practice is required to achieve satisfactory results.

Have realistic expectations. Be realistic in your expectations about family life. No family is absolutely harmonious 100 percent of the time; "happily ever after" is the stuff of Cinderella and "The Brady Bunch." As family therapist Treadway put it in the *Harvard Family Health Letter*, "Real family life is a highly charged activity where people are in close contact and bound to come into conflict from time to time. Expect to have occasional clashes and be willing to confront them. Working through disagreements is ultimately less stressful than trying to ignore them."

Look on the bright side. Juggling multiple roles—wife, mother, working woman—is tough, demanding, and frequently exhausting. But such a lifestyle does have its advantages.

It seems that the more roles a woman takes on, according to researchers at the University of Manitoba, the healthier she's likely to be. These researchers studied 6,000 women and found that "jugglers" were sick less often and reported feeling healthier than women with fewer roles. Cornell University researchers, who studied 313 women over three decades, not only found that the more roles women engage in voluntarily, the better their health as they got older; these researchers also found that the more roles, the higher the self-esteem. Why would that be? "Role involvements give purpose, meaning, and guidance to life," Cornell's Phyllis Moen speculated in *Glamour* magazine. Added Faye Crosby, Ph.D., a professor of psychology at Smith College, having multiple roles "inoculates" women against depression.

Backing this up, a University of Montreal study of 1,123 women with professional careers in medicine, law, engineering, and accounting found that professional single women and married women without children were not as happy with their lives as the married women with children. Another study found that single women with no children have a higher risk of suicide than married women, and the risk of suicide among married women decreases in direct correlation to the number of children they have.

Finally, Wellesley researchers found that mothers (as well as childless women with partners) were much less anxious and depressed than single women without children when the quality of their working life declined—say, because of a demotion or a looming layoff. According to Wellesley psychologist Rosalind Barnett, "Women with family roles have several potential sources of rewards, such as helping others and having authority to make decisions, whereas women without family roles must find rewards at work or suffer the consequences."

In a nutshell: we may have dark circles, but the eyes above them are probably shining.

CHAPTER NINE

THE GREAT DIVIDE

The Incredible Change in Perspective Almost All Mothers Experience

In February 1993, Madeline, then four, began to wear an adhesive-bandage–like eye patch for a few months because our ophthalmologist wanted to make the vision in the unpatched eye as strong as the vision in the patched eye without the aid of glasses (this is achievable only in children under age seven). On the way home from the doctor's office on the first day Madeline wore the patch, we stopped at the library. She was disoriented, she couldn't see very well, and the patch itched, but she was very brave and uncomplaining about it. I was so proud of her.

And then, just as we were about to enter the library, two boys about nine years old came out. One of them pointed at my daughter and laughed. "Look !" he said to his friend. "A one-eyed Martian!"

I found myself whirling around. "How *dare* you make fun of her!" I nearly shrieked. "How would you like it if everyone pointed and laughed at you and called you fat and ugly?"

Both boys were rendered speechless. I pulled my daughter through the library door and slammed it behind me. Then I stood in the library lobby for a minute, just shaking. Finally, I turned to Madeline. "What on earth possessed me to say something so mean?"

I debated for a long time about including that anecdote in this book because it makes me, a person who's written hundreds of words about raising children's self-esteem, look so horrible. In the end, however, I just had to use it, because it is such a perfect example of one of the most profound psychological changes of motherhood. When your child is threatened—and I guess my own experience proves that the threat can be physical or psychological—it is as if pure, primitive, animal instinct takes over. You become a fierce she-bear protecting her cub. It's this instinct that's behind those stories you hear about 120-pound women lifting full-sized Buicks off their children. And it's this instinct that made Ellie Nesler (in a case that was making major headlines in California as I wrote these words) shoot dead the smirking man who was about to be tried for molesting Nesler's young son.

Crossing the great divide into motherhood will change the way you look at the world and the way you *react* to the world in a number of other enormous ways. Some examples:

"Mother to the World"

Motherhood will turn you into a "mother to the world." You will never again be able to hear or read about a tragedy that has befallen a child or about pain that a child is enduring without superimposing your own child in that child's place and/or feeling deep, heart-wrenching empathy for his mother, even if the mother isn't mentioned. For five years now, since Madeline was born, I cannot bear to read any account of child abuse. If I happen to see a headline like "Boyfriend arrested in toddler death" in my morning paper, my eyes fly as if burned to the opposite side of the page.

"Even *Dumbo* and *Bambi* become unendurable," a friend agreed. "And I absolutely refuse to see *Cape Fear*, because there's supposedly a scene where the daughter is threatened with rape in front of the mother." Said another friend, "It would be interesting to find out how many women who are mothers have seen the movie *Sophie's Choice* more than once. I'm willing to bet the answer is zero."

One mother told me she found her maternal feelings extending even to the privileged Chelsea Clinton. "Interestingly, when I was in my twenties, I used to laugh when people made cracks about Amy Carter's looks," this woman said. "But now that I'm a mother, when I hear the same kind of jokes about Chelsea Clinton I get so infuriated I feel tears in my eyes." She's not the only one. When the *Los Angeles Times* printed an article shortly before Bill Clinton's inauguration about Chelsea Clinton and some of the jokes people were making about her, the paper got several angry letters from women, presumably mothers. "It's one thing to show how children's lives change when they are elevated to public scrutiny," wrote Karen Shortridge, "but it is quite another to republish remarks that are hurtful and degrading. Children are not fair game. They need our protection." I remember that I myself fervently hoped that the Clintons had not spent the weekend the article was printed in their Santa Barbara vacation home, where Chelsea would have had easy access to the *L.A. Times.*

Motherhood will alter your political views. Being a mother to the world in combination with the fiercely protective she-bear feelings you have for your own child can radically alter your political views, as well. "My husband says motherhood has turned me into a right-wing nut," said my friend Rachel, naming as a prime example the fact that while she was opposed to the death penalty before she became a mother, she's now solidly in favor of it.

I heard that particular change of heart from mother after mother, including one who said she had actively protested against the death penalty before she gave birth. "When Robert Alton Harris was scheduled to become the first person to be put to death in California in twenty-five years, I wrote reams of letters to newspapers about how 'barbaric' capital punishment was," she said. "Then I had my own son. Now I knew all along that Harris had said to one of the boys he killed, 'Stop crying and die like a man.' But it wasn't until Jason was born that reading that quote made me absolutely livid with rage. The way I feel now is that gas was too good for that guy. If by some miracle Harris came back to life and I had the opportunity to strangle him, I would do it."

Another mom told me that a few days after Ellie Nesler "took aim and bestowed the death penalty" on her son's alleged molester in a California courtroom, a family reunion the mom attended exploded into a raging debate over the case. "The sides were split cleanly down motherhood lines," she said. "On the one side were all of the men plus the women who weren't mothers. They all spouted variations of 'The man deserved his day in court' or 'The penalty for molesting a child is not death.' The motherhood side was split into factions: the moms who said 'Good shootin', Ellie' and the supposedly liberal ACLU types like me, who were *thinking* 'Good shootin', Ellie' but primly said 'I don't condone what she did, but I have to admit I'm glad there's one less monster preying on children in this world.' "

Other Changes in Perspective

Motherhood will change the way you view our culture. Once you have the responsibility of molding a mind, of helping to fill a clean and innocent "blank slate," you will cease to be "live and let live" and become hypercritical of the way our culture celebrates such things as sex, violence, and materialism. One of my friends calls this the "Tipper Gore Phenomenon." "In the mid-1980s, before we had children, it was something of a sport among my group of friends to heap scorn on Tipper Gore for her efforts to get warning labels put on records with graphically sexual or violent lyrics," she explains it. "But in 1992, when Al Gore was running for vice president—and we had all become parents—you heard not a peep among any of us against Tipper. Instead, we all loudly lauded Al and Tipper's commitment to the environment. Once you become a parent, you hear Ice T in an entirely different way."

That same friend is currently boycotting Oliver Stone movies. She read an article in *Premiere* magazine in which the writer asked several prominent film directors if they thought Hollywood should censor itself by cutting down on the amount of violence in the movies. Most of the directors agreed, my friend said, and made comments to the effect that they don't allow their own children to see the movies they make. Oliver Stone, however, saw no need for censorship. "He sounds very irresponsible," she said. "This would not have fazed me before I had my children, but it's terribly important to me now."

Said another mother: "Before I had my children, that

camel the one cigarette company uses in its ads was just a harmless, goofy-looking cartoon character. Now I see him as an evil seducer of children. No kidding."

My own personal motherhood crusade (and one that I believe my extended family laughs at behind my back) has been against fairy tales in which a handsome prince comes along at the end to rescue the girl and make her live happier ever after. Pardon me while I put my feminist cap on, but I believe such tales give little girls unreasonable expectations about marriage while ignoring the fact that girls have their own talents and power to change their lives. I find Cinderella particularly offensive because that story not only does all of the above, it also delivers the messages that the prettiest girl is the *best* girl (to say nothing of its glorification of small feet!) and that relationships between women are primarily competitive and spiteful. After Madeline received the book *Cinderella* on her second birthday, I threw it away and she never even missed it. (By now, she knows about Cinderella anyway, of course. She saw Disney's animated version at a friend's house and came home rhapsodizing about it. It infuriates her when, like a mean big sister instead of a mommy, I refer to it as "Cindersmella." This will probably all backfire on me someday, and she'll end up marrying England's Prince William!)

Motherhood will give you entrée into the biggest and oldest sorority in the world. Anna Quindlen, the *New York Times* columnist, has called ours "the sisterhood of motherhood," with "a set of small handprints executed in fingerpaint" as our coat of arms.

Especially in the first few months after your baby's birth, you will look at every woman with children and think appreciatively, "*She* went through that, too." Even if you and your mother or your sister (who now has kids of her own) never got along, you will suddenly have one very big facet of your life in common with theirs.

As long as she, too, is a mother, you will never again need a conversational ice breaker with another woman. You will find yourself breezily chatting about sore nipples with a complete stranger in the supermarket checkout line. You may, in fact, find it extremely difficult *not* to discuss your children with a fellow mother. A couple of summers ago when I was in the final stages of writing a book, I had the chance to see the book's editor for one hour in New York before my plane left. We spent the entire hour talking about our kids. It wasn't until I was about to hop into a taxi that she asked "How's the book going?" I said "Great!" Then we went our separate ways. Later, we cracked up about that.

I noticed for the first time at a recent party at which all of us were about the same age that not only did men and women split into separate, sexually segregated conversational groups but that the women split yet again into mother and nonmother groups. "The things that make your life harder are the same" is the way a friend explained this, "so even if you're not talking about kids you naturally group together."

As a member of the sorority, you will probably find yourself favoring your fellow members. For example, as a journalist, I have personally gotten women who had made news—news that had nothing to do with motherhood or children—to talk to me when they wouldn't talk to any other journalist, simply because I, too, am a mother.

And you'll find yourself almost automatically taking the side of your fellow mother in a dispute. One woman told me, for example, that she did a complete turnabout on the infamous case of Mary Beth Whitehead (the surrogate mother who gave birth to "Baby M") after her own child was born. "Before Nicole, I was on the Sterns's side," she said. "I remember grimacing at Mary Beth whenever I'd see her on the television news and saying to my husband, 'A contract is a contract.' Now that I can imagine what it must feel like to lose your child, I wish I could steal that baby back for Mary Beth!"

I underwent a similar conversion as I was rereading one of my most cherished childhood books, *Anne Frank: The Diary of a Young Girl*, shortly after Madeline's birth. In a scene in that book, Anne's mother comes to tuck her in, and Anne refuses to let her. As usual, Anne wants her father to do the honors. Saying something like "Love can't be forced," Anne's mother leaves the room with tears in her eyes. Now I have read that book probably every other year since I was ten years old, and that scene didn't faze me in the least until Madeline was born. After that, I found myself *weeping* over that page and saying aloud, "Oh, Anne, how could you be so cruel to her?"

I related that anecdote to one of my friends, and she said she'd experienced a similar change of attitude in regard to the mother in one of her favorite books—Herman Wouk's *Marjorie Morningstar*. "Before my daughter was born, I saw Mrs. Morganstern as overbearing, overprotective, and meddlesome," my friend said. "Now my overriding feeling is that she simply always had Marjorie's best interests at heart and that Marjorie didn't appreciate her enough!"

So we're loyal, yes, but we can be equally as critical and condemning of a mother who betrays the membership. For example (and to keep this discussion in a literary vein) I have another friend who was a passionate devotee of the poems and other writings of the brilliant and tortured Sylvia Plath. "She was absolutely my heroine—until I had a baby," this friend said. "I knew all along that when Plath committed suicide she had two children under the age of five and that those kids were asleep in another room of the apartment when she stuck her head in the oven and turned the gas on. But the selfishness of that act didn't hit me, Sylvia Plath did not come crashing down from her pedestal, till I became a mother myself. I just found it incomprehensible that she could leave her babies. As a sort of symbolic protest, I took *The Bell Jar*, her autobiographical novel, out of the book shelf next to my bed where I keep my favorite books, and I put it in the attic."

Finally, my friend Rachel brought up the point that many of us "have a wicked desire to get everyone else into the sorority," as she put it. In other words, there's a conspiracy among us to convince other women to become mothers, too. As Rachel explained, "It's like talking a friend into going on a scary ride and knowing she's not really up to it and will pee her pants, but dammit, you need company. You need someone to hold onto. Part of it is evangelical, too. You know it's changed your life in these wonderful ways. So you push it like a twelve-step program. And you consciously take care not to disclose the negatives—like sleep deprivation!"

Other mothers have a new respect for women who choose *not* to have children. Once you know how difficult motherhood is, even if you love it, it's easier to understand how someone could choose not to become a mother. While for most women the benefits of motherhood far outweigh the negatives, some women are brutally honest with their friends. "I don't sugarcoat a thing," said one mother of a toddler. "It's the right choice for me, but I know from experience how frustrating it can be even if it's what you *want* to be doing. Heaven help the mom who's doing it just because everyone else does!"

***Motherhood will make you much more aware of your
own mortality.*** The very best example I can give to illus-
trate this is the fact that several women I interviewed told
me that they were never afraid to fly until they had children. "The day after that PSA flight crashed over San
Diego in 1978, I flew on PSA without a qualm" said a
mother who flies frequently on business. "I sat next to this
woman who was just terrified, and I remember saying
something callous and glib like 'Why worry? When your
number's up, your number's up.' Well, since I had my son,
I'm terrified in the air, too. During every second that we're
landing or taking off, and especially during turbulence, I'm
just sweating bullets and thinking 'Who will take care of
him if I die? Who will love him? Will he even remember
me?' This sounds strange, but the only time I'm not afraid
to fly is when he's flying with me—because if I should die,
so will he. At least we'll be together."

Motherhood will make you paranoid. In other words,
you will not just worry about your own mortality. To quote
a dad on this subject: "Every illness you scoffed at as a kid
becomes the bubonic plague when *your* kid gets it," wrote
Scott Lafee in the *San Diego Union-Tribune*. "Every
sneeze, every cough becomes a dark and ominous harbin-
ger. The color of nasal discharge becomes an object of
intense study."

Robin Abcarian, a new mother and columnist for the
Los Angeles Times, recently confessed that while she was
once the "Empress of Easy Going," motherhood has
turned her into the "Queen of Queasy." "Oh, sure, I
fantasize about everyday disasters—choking, falling, and
drowning accidents," she wrote. "But I try to conserve my
energy for contemplation of the truly catastrophic. (This, as
any mentally unbalanced new parent can tell you, is a

form of insurance. If you worry about something really bizarre, it can't possibly happen.)" One of the "truly catastrophic" events Abcarian worries about? That a plane might plummet out of the sky onto the bassinet as her baby naps.

Motherhood will change your idea of what makes for happiness. I am writing this three days after my family returned from a weekend at one of southern California's most famous resorts. The restaurant there is considered one of the best in the state, and as a thank-you for something my husband did, we enjoyed exquisite food, fine wine, good conversation, a spectacular sunset, and even a baby-sitter on the house. Before Madeline was born, this meal would have been what tickled me the most about the weekend. Instead, the memory that makes me happiest is of Steve suddenly rearing up from the bottom of the pool, sputtering and snarling like a sea monster, and of Madeline bursting into peals of helpless laughter no matter how many times he did this.

Singer Amy Grant expressed this change in perspective in terms of Christmas: "When my kids ask me what I want for Christmas, I say what my grandmother used to say," she told *Target the Family* magazine. 'All I want is to be with you guys, to wake up and see your smiling faces and kiss the backs of your necks. That's better than anything I could unwrap in a package.' I used to hate it when she said that. Now it's exactly how I feel."

Motherhood will loosen your inhibitions. Years before I had my own baby, my sister Sally told me she lost her modesty forever after the thirty-hour–plus labor and birth of her first child. When I asked her why, she sent me an Erma Bombeck column by way of explanation. In it, Bombeck proposes that the entrance of every delivery room in the country should carry a sign reading "Here Enters the Last Modest Woman on the Face of the Earth." As Bombeck put it, "There is a stream of men we have never seen before who whip in and out of our hospital rooms like they are caught in a revolving door. They invade our bare chests with stethoscopes and throw back the sheets to 'take a look at what we have here.' They thumb, probe, squeeze, and push on every part of our bodies. They interrupt our baths to inquire about our irregularities and watch us struggle with hospital gowns that are too small to set a cocktail glass on." After all that, Bombeck concludes, it's nothing to sit at the breakfast table with your robe open.

Another mom told me she began to lose her modesty even before her baby was born. "When you're pregnant, it's as if your body becomes public property," she said. "You get used to perfect strangers walking up and patting your tummy or asking you how much weight you've put on."

A friend, Marnie, told me having her own kid has made her much less inhibited when dealing with *other* people's kids. "Our house is on a popular route home from the elementary school," Marnie told me. "Before I had my baby, kids used to run through the flower bed in our front yard, and I'd just watch them from behind the curtain and silently fume. I'd think, 'Oh, God, if I go out there and yell at them, they're going to think I'm some sort of witch lady.' Even when I did work up the courage to bleat a complaint out the window, they'd just ignore it. Nowadays, if any kid dares to set foot in that flower bed, I hustle right out, read the riot act, and he never tries it again."

Her new ability to do this has "mother to the world" overtones. Deep down, most mothers feel it's their duty not just to keep an eye on all kids—"Are you lost, honey?"—

but to keep all kids in line, as well. But Marnie believes what's *really* behind her new, confident manner is the "authoritative 'mommy tone' that creeps into your voice box and takes up permanent residence there once your child learns to walk," she said. "Kids, all kids, really do take more heed of it."

Marnie feels her new authoritativeness has also helped her in situations that don't involve children. "For example, we often patronize a crowded neighborhood ice cream shop where the owners, much to my frustration, have a take-a-number system but don't use it," Marnie said. "It used to be I'd suffer in silence when someone came into the store after I did, pushed up to the counter, and got waited on out of turn. Nowadays, I have absolutely no problem pushing up next to the aggressive little cheater and announcing in no uncertain terms, 'Excuse me, but I was next!'"

Along these same lines, model Christie Brinkley says motherhood has helped her overcome her shyness and her difficulty in dealing with strangers. "I have to call up other moms to set up play dates," Brinkley told *Ladies' Home Journal* in regard to her daughter Alexa. "I have to set an example for her, because she's terribly shy, too."

Motherhood will change the way you view your parents. You will see your parents differently. Especially your mother. It will give you a new appreciation of her, a new bond because of what you suddenly have in common: the raising of children.

Charlotte, a friend, told me that before she had her son, she spent two years in therapy "mainly exploring issues concerning my mother. At the end of that therapy, I felt everything was pretty much resolved, that I'd let go of all my angry, frustrated feelings. But it wasn't until I had my son that I *really* let them go. Once you have a child, you realize how exhausted and self-sacrificing your parents were. You can't focus on their mistakes anymore; in fact, you're kind of grateful that they *weren't* perfect parents because, Lord knows, *you* aren't (or at least *I'm* not). Also, although I've made different choices, such as not to spank, I realize that my parents were raising kids at a different time, under different advice."

My friend Rachel believes that another reason women often become closer to their mothers after becoming mothers themselves "is that you suddenly need her in ways you never before needed older women." When Rachel's second child, John Phillip, had bad diarrhea, for example, Rachel called her mother in a panic: "What can I do? You're not supposed to give babies Pepto-Bismol." Do what my grandmother always did, her mother replied: boil rice and then feed John some of the water after it cools. It worked like a charm.

"I also remember calling my parents a few weeks after John Phillip was born because my husband was working late and I just needed to talk to someone who had been there, who had been as bone-tired and completely drained as I was at that moment," Rachel said. "Before I had my children, I never would have turned to my mother and father in such an honest, humble, needy way. They really do become your peers instead of your parents."

Motherhood may change what you look for in friends.
Specifically, you will find you really need friends who are also the mothers of small children—at first because all you'll want to talk about is baby-baby-baby (see "Possessed!" in Chapter 7) and in later years so that you can commiserate, compare notes, and give your kids a chance to play together.

When Madeline was born, not a single other woman in my crowd had children. Most of them, in fact, weren't even married. Desperate for mommy talk, I used to make the rounds of all the local parks, hunting down potential friends. And I found them. I met Rachel at a park when both of us shouted "Madeline!" and then stared at each other in amazement (and we later discovered we not only had daughters with the same name but also husbands named Stephen Alan). She had been similarly hungry for mommy friends. In fact, one morning, out for a lonely neighborhood walk with her Madeline in a stroller, Rachel—hearing a baby cry as she passed a house—strode up the front walk, rapped on the screen door, and called out, "Is there a mother in there?"

In the first couple of years of Madeline's life, as long as a woman had a toddler in tow and didn't say "he don't" instead of "he doesn't," we were in business; I had myself a friend. Once past those scary first years, however, motherhood ceases to be a unifying factor solely on its own. I eventually drifted away from my new mom friends who hated the idea of reading for pleasure, then from those who didn't think "Seinfeld" was funny, and so on. Still, most of my closest friends today are mothers, and our friendships are as deep and rich, our conversations as broad and all-encompassing, as those I had with friends before Madeline was born. And friendships between moms have two extra benefits: one, you have an additional, limitless topic of conversation (raising children) and, two, your kids can entertain each other during the visit instead of hanging around and whining "When are we going home?" or asking "What's a diaphragm?" like they do when you're with someone who *doesn't* have kids.

"Once you have children," said my friend Glenda, "when you meet new people you automatically award them ten extra points on the 'potential friend?' rating scale if they happen to be parents."

Motherhood will change the way you feel about work. We touched upon feelings about working in Chapter 7 in the section "The End of Maternity Leave." For most women (and many men, too) parenthood often pushes one's career down a rung or two on the ladder of priorities. As Barbara Dafoe Whitehead recently wrote in the scholarly publication *Family Affairs*, "More and more parents of young children are realizing that work life and family life conflict, that time is scarcer than money, and that time and attention are the chief currency of family life and the well being of children."

For some women, motherhood pushes career off the ladder altogether, at least temporarily. A woman I know who spent a decade (including her son's first two years) in a job she adored—she was the children's librarian at a local library—recently quit. "It was hard enough to leave him when he was a baby," she said. "But now he is a little person full of delightful observations of his own, and I am no longer willing to let a babysitter be the chief beneficiary of all that."

Motherhood will make you less selfish, less self-centered. The most profound example of this: probably for the first time in your life, you will find that you would unquestionably and instantaneously give up your own life to save that of someone else—your child.

Another example: I myself first discovered that motherhood had made me much less egocentric the way I discover most things: through a book. Dragging poor Anne Frank into this chapter again, I'll mention the epilogue in *Anne Frank: The Diary of a Young Girl*, in which the editor describes in stark but moving terms how Anne, alone in a filthy bed in a Nazi concentration camp, finally dies of typhus. Every time I used to read that description, I'd picture myself under such circumstances and would dissolve in tears. These days, the passage still makes me weep; but instead of picturing myself, I picture *Madeline* in that bed.

These are pretty dramatic examples. But motherhood will make you less selfish and less self-centered in small, everyday ways, as well. "Days of Our Lives" star Deidre Hall provided one such example from *her* everyday life about a year after she adopted a baby. Said Hall in *People* magazine, "My makeup man asked if he could give me a gash on my face [to enhance a story line] and I said okay. Then he said, 'What if it's bleeding? What if it's *oozing?*' And I said, 'It's your job, you do it.' And he said, 'A year ago, you would have said okay, a little cut, but make it on the cheekbone. You know, I think you're finally over yourself.'"

Motherhood will change the way you view your community. When you don't have children, you can remain completely socially isolated from your neighbors if you so desire. That changes radically, however, once you have children. You need to know these people because your child will be playing in or near their homes. Suddenly, a neighbor's own child-rearing practices become a prime concern. Do they give their toddler soft drinks? Do they allow their four-year-old to watch *Pretty Woman* and *Terminator 2*? And what about their own proclivities? Do they collect guns? Or pornography? Do they have criminal records? And do they have fourteen- or fifteen-year-old daughters who babysit?

"I remember my husband and I used to laugh about this

old man down the street who was known for walking around his house and backyard stark naked," a woman told me. "He wasn't a pervert; he simply sometimes forgot to put clothes on. But the minute we had Sam, I stopped seeing him as a harmless old crackpot. His whole house took on a sort of sinister glow in my mind, and I remember saying almost hysterically to my husband one day, 'We have to do something about Mr. X!' " (And they did. They moved.)

You also need your neighbors—both those with kids and those without—to know your child, as well, because you will depend on them to keep an eye out for your child; to intervene, say, if they spot a stranger approaching your child.

For your child's sake you will be forced to interact with people you never would have chosen to deal with on your own, either because your kid is best friends with their kid or because they, too, got suckered into volunteering to work the dunk-a-dad booth at the school Halloween carnival.

And when you go to buy a bigger house, whole sections of your city—areas you once coveted because they're, say, much closer to the ocean or to your office—will simply cease to exist because the schools there are crummy or the streets too busy.

Motherhood will change the way you think about the future. For many of us, "the future" when we were not parents meant next weekend or next fall. Once you have a child, the future becomes the rest of that child's life, plus her child's life, as well. Suddenly, who the next president will be really matters. You become passionate about issues that you merely felt strongly about before you became pregnant, issues such as abortion and the environment. I know many mothers my age who became actively involved in politics for the first time during the elections of 1992. Two of these women confessed that they had never even bothered to vote preparenthood.

"Suddenly, something as simple as whether to throw your Snapple bottle away in the trash can at the park or to haul it home and put it in your recycling bin becomes an issue," a woman told me. "I know it sounds terribly corny and righteous, but you really do become concerned about the kind of world we're going to leave behind, because your own child will have to deal with it."

CHAPTER TEN

FULL SPEED AHEAD

Getting the Most
out of Your New Body and New Life

At a party not too long ago, a few of us were looking at an old *Life* magazine. The cover story was about Marilyn Monroe, and an eleven-year-old girl piped up, *"She* was a movie star? But she has a *humongous* butt!"

This incident got me marveling at the ironic fact that, while women have come so far in so many areas since Marilyn's heyday, the standard of beauty we're held to has gotten increasingly more rigid and more impossible to achieve. First, along came Twiggy, ushering in what's been called "the tyranny of slender," this seemingly endless dictate that women must be thin—and preferably tall, too—in order to be considered attractive. Then, in the 1980s, the fitness boom gave birth to another requirement: a taut, firm, muscular body. And now here we are in the 1990s, and Madison Avenue has decided that since we're all supposedly "cocooning," turning our attention back to hearth and home, we must be obviously, gloriously femi-nine, as well. The result? Nowadays, the ideal female in the

United States is a tall, slender hardbody with big boobs.

Is it any wonder that so many women hate their bodies? Look at the results of recent studies:

• 95 percent of "normal-sized women" overestimate their body size.

• 80 percent of women in the U.S. think they're overweight, while only 25 percent actually are.

• 74 percent of women have negative feelings about their thighs; the stomach is in second place with a 65 percent disapproval rating.

• While the average U.S. woman is five feet, four inches and weighs 142 pounds, she wishes she was five feet, six inches and weighed 129 pounds.

• Women are ten times more likely than men to suffer eating disorders such as anorexia and bulimia.

There can be no doubt, if you read Dear Abby (the headline of her column on the day I am writing this is "Mother's 'Baby Fat' Has Ruined Her Life") and listen in on the conversation of any group of new mothers, that the first year or two postpartum are particularly hard for body haters. Not only do you have those beauties on the billboards to contend with, you're also comparing yourself to the you of nine months ago—who may not have been a tall, slender hardbody with big boobs but who almost certainly weighed less than today's you. On top of that, you no longer have the time/energy/money/all of the above to buy hope from the industry that's sprung up and made billions because U.S. women hate their bodies: the diet centers, the fitness clubs, the plastic surgeons.

So what do you do if you've lost all your baby fat and you still aren't satisfied? What do you do if you're grateful for the fact that your menstrual cramps will never again be as bad and that your breast cancer risks have dropped but you still hate your new, smaller, saggier breasts; you hate the stretch marks and the looser, flabbier feel of the skin on your stomach; *in short, you hate the way your body looks more than ever?*

There comes a time to stop trying to change or hoping to change your body and to start changing the way you *feel* about it. A poor body image has a much bigger effect on your life than just keeping you off the beach. According to body-image researcher Thomas Cash, Ph.D., of Old Dominion University, body image constitutes a whopping 25 to 33 percent of a person's sense of confidence. A poor body image can contribute to both depression and low self-esteem, and obsessing about your physical flaws also uses up energy that could better be used for creativity, productivity, and self-realization, according to Marcia Germaine Hutchinson, a Boston psychologist and author of *Transforming Body Image: Learning to Love the Body You Have* (Crossing Press). Body hatred can also impact your physical health—leading to stringent dieting that can cause a host of problems or even to disorders such as compulsive eating (to numb insecure feelings), bulimia, or anorexia.

There's a reason early motherhood is an especially good time to change your mind's body image: Children pick up most of their attitudes at home, and all of us (particularly those with daughters) should commit ourselves to not raising another generation of slaves to Slim-Fast. "You do not know devastation until your three-year-old daughter looks up from her potty chair and announces in her baby voice, 'My thighs are too fat,' " a woman told me. "Believe me, I got my consciousness raised real fast that day."

Changing the way you view your body image is not an easy process, especially when you've had twenty, twenty-five, or thirty years of conditioning in the wrong direction. I've gathered, however, a handful of ideas from mothers, psychologists, and other experts that have worked for others and that should at least get you on the right road—if not to *loving* your body, at least to accepting and appreciating it.

Get real. One of the most comforting and eye-opening improve-your-body-image exercises is to discreetly scrutinize a group of women, women in your own age group, in your everyday life so that your idea of what real women look like becomes less dependent on the bodies you see in ads and on the cover of *People*. Do some "girl watching" on a bench at the mall or (even better) observe women in a state of semi-undress, such as in a locker room or a store's communal dressing room. Here in California, the legendary Nordstrom department store rigs up the latter, whenever it has one of its famous semiannual sales. I remember Madeline, at age four, getting her own little consciousness raised in such a Nordstrom communal dressing room. Turning to me wide-eyed as I shrugged into a new suit jacket, she exclaimed, "Mommy, everybody's body is so *different!*" Until then, I realized, Barbie and I were her only role models for what a partially naked adult woman's body looks like. (Just don't stare at the women in the dressing room like Madeline did!)

Similarly, some women begin to feel better about their bodies when they find out that their weight is within the normal and healthy range for their height. (Remember, while 80 percent of U.S. women think they are overweight, only 25 percent actually are.) Insurance tables are one place to get this information—ask your physician or insurance agent. *The World Almanac and Book of Facts*, widely available at bookstores and libraries, offers a chart of the average weight of Americans by height, age, and gender.

By the same token, you can quiet an obsession with how much body fat you have by getting a body-fat test to determine if you're within the normal range. If you're not athletic, 28 to 30 percent body fat is considered normal; 22 to 25 percent means you're relatively slender and physically fit. Health clubs, sports medicine clinics, health fairs, YMCAs and YWCAs, and many doctors offer body-fat testing, with fees generally ranging from ten dollars to forty-five dollars. The traditional methods of body-fat testing are hydrostatic weighing (you get into a tank of water, and the tester notes how much water is displaced) and with an instrument called a caliper that measures the thickness of your skin in various areas. Newer methods employ harmless electrical current and infrared light.

Finally, it's important to realize that much of the beauty you see on television and in magazines is not natural. Many actresses and models resort to starvation and/or extreme exercise regimens (actress Julianne Phillips of TV's "Sisters," for example, disclosed that she does *six thousand abdominal crunches a week!*), and/or their beauty has been created surgically or photographically. No one knows about the latter better than I, the wife of a professional photographer. I wish every woman in the United States could watch a photographer's studio session with a model, just to witness the miracles the photographer can perform with lighting, lenses, and filters. And should a flaw somehow slip through onto film, there's a second string ready and waiting: photo retouchers. The stars you see on the covers of women's magazines always get it in writing that retouching will be performed to their satisfaction. Furthermore, photographs of models are often trimmed with scissors, according to Naomi Wolf, who wrote *The Beauty Myth* (Morrow).

She also reported that a computer graphics machine called Scitex alters just about every fashion or glamour photo that the public sees.

Savor praise. Start a list of every compliment people make about your appearance. To restore your confidence, take this list out and read it over very slowly on days when you feel particularly insecure about your looks.

On this same subject, when you stop negating expressions of praise from others, you begin to stop negating them to yourself. In other words, when you're paid a compliment, don't say something negative like "This old thing?" Just say thanks.

Get a second opinion. If you're not out and about enough to collect compliments, ask a close friend or your husband what he or she thinks is physically attractive about you. Then try to give this second opinion as much weight as you do your own harsh judgments about yourself. After all, it's coming from another person (besides yourself) who looks at you every day.

Make friends, or at least a truce, with your mirror. Many women who hate their bodies hide them not just from their husbands (no lovemaking till the lights are out, for example) but from themselves, as well. Spend five minutes a day standing nude in front of a mirror just looking at yourself. You'll start feeling more comfortable with your body as looking at it becomes routine.

While you're at it, admire the body parts you've always liked. In her best-selling book *Revolution from Within: A Book of Self-Esteem* (Little, Brown), Gloria Steinem said she's always been proud of the hands she inherited from her father. She went on to say that she makes a conscious effort to expand these positive, empowering feelings of approval to the rest of her body, as well.

You can, too. Counteract every negative judgment that comes to mind. To revise an old maxim, if you can't say something nice, then at least say something neutral. For example, if you find yourself beginning to think "My upper arms are flabby and ugly" and can't make yourself say "My arms are beautiful," go with "My arms are strong."

Live in the now. The translation of the New Age–ese "live in the now" is: get rid of all of those old clothes in your closet that are too small and that you're saving for the day you lose weight. Those clothes are serving as nothing more than reproachful reminders. They do not represent the you of today, the woman who has changed in so many wonderful ways. To say nothing of the fact that they are probably also out of style.

Have at least one "bad hair day" outfit. Every woman has one dress or outfit that looks fabulous on her. It fits great, is a favorite color, and always draws compliments. Wear it on days that you feel especially insecure about your looks. Resist fashion if necessary and concentrate on building a collection of such feel-good outfits so you can feel good about the way you look every day.

Look at photographs and paintings of women in earlier eras. Flip through old *Life* magazines, for example, or visit an art museum for evidence of just how much the definition of beauty changes over the years. It's a very faddish and fickle business. For example, in the fourteenth and fifteenth centuries, "beautiful" women shaved off their eyebrows plus two or three inches of their hairline at the crown for an "egghead" effect. Today's fad (tall-thin-muscular-busty), too, shall pass—in our own or at least in our daughters' lifetimes, let us hope. Future generations will pull late twentieth-century magazine advertisements out of time capsules and shake their heads in wonder: "Why would they photograph ill, starving women?"

Build up your self-esteem in other areas of your life. The confidence that building your "out-of-body" self-esteem engenders can spill over and make you feel more confident about your looks, too. "I am a stay-at-home mom who weighs 250 pounds," a woman told me, "and I found that once I got involved in some extracurricular activities— I joined my church choir and became a Girl Scout leader—I not only had less time to dwell on my body, the fact that I'm fat also began to be crowded out by other factors when I think about who I am. I am no longer just a fat mother. I am also a woman who brings enjoyment to hundreds of people every Sunday morning and who is helping a dozen ten-year-old girls learn valuable life skills and serve their community."

Evaluate your best friends. Picture each of your closest friends and ask yourself: What do I like best about this person? It may surprise you to realize that looks are almost never at the top of the list. What we usually value most are features like "her sympathetic ear" or "his ability to make me laugh." This exercise can help you understand that not only are looks not everything, they often don't count at all.

Pamper yourself. When your body feels good physically, it's easier to feel better about it mentally. Get a massage. Soak in fragrant bubbles. Coat your feet with Vaseline and wear socks to bed. "My one and only luxury is a weekly manicure," said a mother with long, red acrylics. "To me, it works like magic. When my hands look pretty, I feel pretty all over."

Get professional help. Especially if your body image has you mired in depression or is otherwise interfering with your life in a big way, you should seek professional help. A *cognitive* therapist, in particular, can help you change negative thought patterns. There are even some therapists who specialize in treating women with body-image problems. A good way to find one: call an eating disorders clinic (most large hospitals have such clinics) and ask for a referral.

Read an enlightening book on this subject. Like a sudden backlash against the impossible ideal, several good books about (or partially about) the poor body image of the U.S. woman have been published in just the last few years. From them you can learn in greater detail how you came to hate your body and what you can do to change that. A recommended reading list:

• *Bodylove: Learning to Like Our Looks and Ourselves,* by Rita Freedman, Ph.D. (Harper & Row).

• *The Beauty Myth: How Images of Beauty Are Used Against Women,* by Naomi Wolf (Morrow).

• *Body Traps: Breaking the Binds That Keep You from Feeling Good About Yourself,* by Judith Rodin, Ph.D. (Morrow).

• *Transforming Body Image: Learning to Love the Body You Have,* by Marcia Germaine Hutchinson, Ph.D. (Crossing Press).

• *Revolution from Within: A Book of Self-Esteem*, by Gloria Steinem (Little, Brown).

Learn to identify the real triggers for your body hatred. One of the exercises Judith Rodin suggests in *Body Traps* (see list above) is to sit down every night, write out each time that you were critical of your body during the day, and then look for reasons you might have been angry at or disappointed in yourself at the time. Did you lose the courage to complain to your boss about your hours, as you had planned to? Did you argue with your mother? Rodin believes people often blame their bodies when external circumstances are really to blame. She feels that learning to identify what *really* triggered the negative feelings about your body can dissipate those negative feelings.

Declaw your painful feelings. One of the suggestions of Boston psychologist Marcia Germaine Hutchinson (see reading list above) is to draw a nude picture of yourself and circle the parts you don't like. Then write down exactly what you don't like about each part: too big, too small, too lumpy and bumpy, and so on. Hutchinson believes this drains some of the pain from such feelings, since repressed emotions have more power that those that are acknowledged.

Celebrate your body as a miracle maker! Many women gain a new respect—even awe—of their bodies during the pregnancy and childbirth experience. "You go for years carrying around all that reproductive equipment down there, bitching about your periods and doing everything in your power to keep from getting pregnant, and then, when you suddenly decide you *want* to get pregnant, your body forgives you for all the years of caffeine and other abuse and obliges you," is the way a friend put it. "It obligingly sends an egg down the tube at the correct time, gets that egg fertilized, then forms and nourishes a complete little human being. Then, entirely of its own volition, except for a little effort on your part at the very end, it gets that baby out of there. It comes up with a complete source of nutrition. Then it immediately gears up to produce another little miracle, if you want one! I remember lying in my hospital bed holding my baby daughter and wearing a goofy, sappy smile, just thinking about the miracles of the female body."

The trick is to carry that admiration into the months and years that follow the heady glow of childbirth, to use that admiration to quiet those sudden surges of body hatred. Admire your body for giving you the strength you never knew you had to carry a twenty-five–pound toddler in one arm and a twenty-five–pound diaper bag in the other. Admire your body for continuing to function through weeks of sleep deprivation. Admire your body for giving you—the woman who, premotherhood, would abandon her cart in the grocery store rather than wait in a line of more than three people—bottomless stores of patience to answer questions like "Why is the sky blue?" and to just shake your head and smile when a three-block walk to the post office takes forty-five minutes because your toddler or preschooler must stop to smell every rose and inspect every "roly-poly" bug.

Recognize the rewards. Admit it: Doesn't the kid make a little sagging here, a little softness there, and a few extra pounds over yonder worth it? "One summer when my daughter was very young and I finally found the courage to be seen in public in a bathing suit again, we went to a crowded community pool, where she pointed to the stretch marks on my hips and practically shouted, 'Mommy, what are all those white, squiggly snakes?' " a woman told me with a laugh. "I was horribly embarrassed until this older woman smiled at my daughter and said, 'Those lines are to remind your mommy about how very much she wanted you and how very much she loves you.' I thought that was a wonderful thing to say, and in many ways it turned my thinking around. To this day, every time I see those stretch marks, I don't feel revulsion at all. I am just suffused with pride and love for what my body created."

I read that quote to my friend Glenda, and she laughed. "I'm not *that* far along on the road to body love," she said, "but it is true that when I look at my little boy and think about how integral and important he has become to me, how he has made my life so much richer in every way, then the physical trade-offs seem mighty minor. I was no larger than a size 8 for thirty-two years and now I'm a 12 who's given up hope of ever fitting into single digits again. Sometimes I mourn for those spandex days. But if I had the chance to do it all over and I knew in advance that I'd permanently end up a size 12, or a 14—or even a 16—I'd do it again in a flash. An absolute flash."

BODY CHANGES AT A GLANCE

The Body and Its Functions

Abdomen—Skin is likely to be slightly but permanently looser than prepregnancy. Some stretching of muscles and ligaments is permanent, but with exercise having a flat abdomen again is possible (though it may never again be quite as flat as before).

Bladder—Function and position can be changed permanently because of the stretching of the pelvic support system during pregnancy and childbirth. Reduced bladder capacity and/or stress incontinence are possible problems.

Breasts—May shrink up to one cup size per pregnancy because some breast tissue is lost. Some sagging is also unavoidable due to permanent stretching of supportive ligaments.

Cervix—Will be larger and more irregularly shaped than prepregnancy. Changes may result in heavier vaginal discharge.

Eyes—Shape of the cornea typically gets steeper, and tear film decreases during pregnancy. Eyes return to pre-pregnancy state six to nine months after birth (longer for breastfeeders).

Fat and weight—The average pregnant woman gains about 4 kilograms (8.82 pounds) of fat. Much of this can be used to nourish the fetus and breastfeed the baby; however, on average, mothers keep about 5 extra pounds of weight per child.

Feet—A permanent increase of up to one shoe size per pregnancy is possible.

Hair—Becomes thicker and more luxuriant during pregnancy due to extended growing cycle. Shedding, or "resting," phase is consequently extended in the first months after birth. Hair loss peaks at six months postpartum.

Immune system—Pregnancy and childbirth do not appear to affect the immune system in any long-lasting or permanent way.

Labia—Remain softer and fleshier than prebaby.

Menstruation—New hormonal levels may result in a change in the menstrual pattern (e.g., more or fewer days of bleeding, longer or shorter times between periods). Cramping is usually diminished for good.

Perspiration—May be profuse for first six to eight weeks after pregnancy as the body rids itself of excess fluids; increased perspiration rate may last several months.

Rectum—Function and position can be changed permanently, thanks to the stretching of the pelvic support mechanisms. In rare cases, the wall between the vagina and rectum remains relaxed, resulting in difficulty moving the bowels.

Ribs—Lowest three ribs on each side flare out during

pregnancy; they can be pulled back in after pregnancy by strengthening abdominal muscles.

Spine—Pressure from the growing fetus can slightly but permanently alter the curvature of the spine.

Strength, endurance, and fitness levels—With exercise, fitness level can be improved during pregnancy or after; strength often increases after pregnancy; athletic endurance, too, often improves after childbirth.

Teeth—Pregnancy brings higher risk of gingivitis (early gum disease) and gum tumors. Without scrupulous care during pregnancy, gingivitis can become chronic afterward. There is no truth to the myth that the fetus extracts calcium from the teeth.

Uterus—Shrinks twentyfold (from about two pounds to two ounces) in the six weeks after birth, then remains marginally larger and rides lower than prepregnancy.

Vagina—Gradually shrinks down and regains most of its prepregnancy muscle tone in the first two months after birth but will forever remain slightly larger than prepregnancy.

Conditions and Diseases

Acne—Fluctuating hormonal levels can promote breakouts for several months after childbirth.

AIDS—Pregnancy and childbirth have little or no effect on the course of the disease.

Allergies—Pregnancy itself may cause a temporary allergy-like, stuffed-up-nose condition called vasomotor rhinitis of pregnancy; otherwise, pregnancy and childbirth are not believed to alter antibody levels, which are tied to allergies.

Asthma—Asthma will improve in one-third of pregnant

women, worsen in another third, and stay the same in the final third. After pregnancy, the condition usually goes back to the way it was prepregnancy.

Cancer—Having a baby decreases your risks of contracting breast, ovarian, uterine, endometrial, bladder, colon, and brain cancers. A woman's risk of contracting cervical, rectal, and pancreatic cancers apparently aren't affected by her reproductive history. Women who have given birth have a slightly higher risk of contracting kidney cancer.

Chronic fatigue syndrome (CFS)—Tends to improve or even disappear during pregnancy, then usually does not return after childbirth.

Diabetes—Some pregnant women develop a temporary form of diabetes called gestational diabetes mellitus (GDM). A percentage of these women will go on to develop Type II diabetes, a permanent version. Women who are diabetic before pregnancy will see their insulin requirement increase during pregnancy, then return to the prepregnancy level after childbirth. If diabetes is not properly controlled during pregnancy, it can worsen existing diabetes-spawned eye or kidney problems.

Diastasis recti abdominis—A major tear of the band of connective tissue called the *linea alba* that runs down the median line of the abdominal wall and joins the abdominal muscles in the middle. This condition persists after childbirth and may require surgery or corrective exercises.

Endometriosis—Progress of the condition is halted during pregnancy, which is often a permanent "cure."

Gallstones—High hormonal levels make pregnant women more susceptible to gallstones. This susceptibility ends within weeks of childbirth.

Heart disease—Women with multiple pregnancies of five or fewer have a 30 percent higher risk of developing heart disease than a woman who has never been pregnant; six or more pregnancies increase the risk 70 percent. These findings are very new and therefore very tentative.

Hemorrhoids—Pressure on the pelvic floor, expanding blood supply, constipation, and pushing during delivery give 70 percent of pregnant women hemorrhoids. Most hemorrhoids shrink within a few weeks of birth, but the problem often doesn't disappear completely without professional treatment.

Linea nigra—A thin dark line that runs up the center of the abdomen and darkens as pregnancy progresses. Usually disappears within the first six months after childbirth.

Mask of pregnancy—Brownish pigment stains across the forehead, cheeks, and nose due to high hormonal levels during pregnancy. The stains usually disappear within the first six months after delivery but may require help from a dermatologist.

Migraine—Some women get their first-ever migraine during the first trimester of pregnancy. Most migraine sufferers see their headaches decrease or cease entirely during the second and third trimesters. Many women see an increase in the number of migraines suffered— compared to prepregnancy—once menstruation begins again after childbirth.

Moles—Pregnancy can accelerate growth of potentially cancerous moles and cause development of new moles and of cherry angiomas ("blood moles").

Osteoporosis—No significant association has been found between this bone-thinning condition and number of pregnancies or breastfeeding.

Perioral dermatitis—Red rash on chin and around mouth that is often triggered by pregnancy. Requires professional treatment; may reappear periodically for six months to two years.

Premenstrual syndrome (PMS)—Generally worsens with each birth (and with age).

Skin tags—Pregnancy can cause development of these benign growths, officially known as fibroepithelial polyps. They remain after pregnancy.

Spider veins—Elevated estrogen levels make many women susceptible to these fine, dilated blood vessels on the face, neck, chest, hands, and arms. Spider veins tend to disappear after childbirth.

Stretch marks—Color will fade in time, but indentations are probably permanent.

Varicose veins—Pressure on the pelvic floor, expanding blood supply, and constipation give one in four pregnant women varicose veins. They tend to improve after childbirth but don't disappear completely without professional treatment; also, they are exacerbated with each subsequent pregnancy.

Fat, Sodium, and Added Sugars in Foods

Values given in the following charts are averages for typical foods in each category; individual products vary. Fats and sugars are listed by grams; sodium and cholesterol by milligrams. One teaspoon of table sugar equals about four grams. "Sugars" refers to all caloric sweeteners added to foods, not to the sugars that occur naturally in fruit, vegetables, and milk. If no numbers are listed, the amounts of fat, sodium, or added sugars are negligible. All figures were supplied by the U.S.D.A. Human Nutrition Information Service.

Common Foods

Breads, Cereals, Grain Products	Fat	Sodium	Sugars
Bagel (½)	1	150	
Biscuit (one, 1 oz.)	2	200	
Bread (1 slice)	1	150	

Breads (cont.)	Fat	Sodium	Sugars
Cereals, cooked (½ cup)			
Cereals, ready to eat			
Plain (1 oz.)	1	300	2
Sweetened (1 oz.)	1	150	14
Crackers (½ oz.)	3	150	
Croissant (one, 2 oz.)	12	450	2
Danish pastry (one, 2 oz.)	12	200	6
Donut	12	200	10
English muffin (½)	1	150	
Granola (1 oz.)	5	50	8
Muffin (one, 1½ oz.)	5	300	4
Pancake (one, 1 oz.)	2	200	
Pasta (½ cup)			
Rice (½ cup)			

Desserts and Snacks	Fat	Sodium	Sugars
Cake			
Angel food (½ cake)		250	22
Frosted (⅟₁₆ cake)	8	150	32
Cheesecake (⅟₁₂ cake)	18	200	18
Chocolate bar (1 oz.)	9		12
Cookies, commercial (4 cookies)	8	150	12
Corn chips (1 oz.)	9	250	
Gelatin dessert (½ cup)		50	14
Ice cream (½ cup)	7	50	14
Ice milk (½ cup)	3	50	12
Peanut butter (2 tbsp.)	16	150	
Peanuts, unsalted (1 oz.)	14		
Pie, fruit (⅙ of 9-in. pie)	18	500	22
Potato chips (1 oz.)	10	150	
Pretzels (1 oz.)		450	

Desserts (cont.)	*Fat*	*Sodium*	*Sugars*
Sherbet (½ cup)	2	50	28
Soft drink (12 fl. oz.)		50	36
Walnuts, unsalted (1 oz.)	18		

Fruit	*Fat*	*Sodium*	*Sugars*
Avocado (½ medium)	15		
Fruit, canned (½ cup)			
In heavy syrup			20
In own juice			
Fruit, fresh (1 medium)			
Fruit, frozen in syrup (½ cup)			22
Fruit juice (¾ cup)			
Sweetened			20
Unsweetened			
Salad, Waldorf (½ cup)	6	100	2

Meat, Poultry, Fish (cooked)	*Fat*	*Sodium*	*Sugars*
Beef, ground, lean (3 oz.)	15	100	
Beef, trimmed (3 oz.)			
Fattier cuts	14	50	
Lean cuts	7	50	
Bologna (2 oz.)	16	600	
Chicken, breaded and fried (3 oz.)	14	250	
Egg, whole (1 large)	6	50	
Fish (3 oz.)			
Finfish, fresh	2	100	
Shellfish, fresh	1	250	
Tuna, canned in water	2	350	
Frankfurter (2 oz.)	16	600	
Ham, lean, roasted (3 oz.)	8	1,250	

Meat (cont.)	Fat	Sodium	Sugars
Pork, trimmed (3 oz.)			
Fattier cuts	14	50	
Lean cuts	7	50	
Poultry, no skin (3 oz.)			
Dark meat	7	50	
Light meat	3	50	
Sausage, pork (2 oz.)	18	850	

Milk, Yogurt, Cheese	Fat	Sodium	Sugars
Cheese (1½ oz.)			
American, process	14	600	
Cheddar	14	250	
Mozzarella, part skim	8	250	
Swiss	12	100	
Cottage Cheese, 4% fat (½ cup)	4	450	
Milk (1 cup)			
Buttermilk	2	250	
Chocolate, 2% fat	5	150	12
Low-fat, 2%	5	100	
Skim		150	
Whole	8	100	
Shake, chocolate	8	300	52
Yogurt, low-fat (1 cup)			
Flavored	3	150	16
Fruit	2	150	28
Plain	4	150	

Spreads, Dressings, Condiments	Fat	Sodium	Sugars
Barbecue sauce (1 tbsp.)		150	2
Butter, margarine (1 tbsp.)	11	100	
Honey (1 tbsp.)			20

Spreads (cont.)	*Fat*	*Sodium*	*Sugars*
Italian Dressing (1 tbsp.)			
Low-calorie		150	
Regular	9	150	2
Jams and jellies (1 tbsp.)			12
Ketchup (1 tbsp.)		150	2
Mayonnaise (1 tbsp.)	11	100	
Mayonnaise-type salad dressing			
(1 tbsp.)	5	100	2
Molasses (1 tbsp.)			20
Mustard (1 tbsp.)		150	2
Olives, green (4 medium)	2	300	
Pickle, dill (1 medium)		950	
Relish, sweet (1 tbsp.)		150	2
Soy sauce (1 tbsp.)		1,050	
Sugar (1 tbsp.)			12
Syrup (1 tbsp.)			20
Vegetable oil (1 tbsp.)	14		
Worcestershire sauce (1 tbsp.)		200	

Vegetables	*Fat*	*Sodium*	*Sugars*
Fresh or frozen vegetables (½ cup)			
Potatoes, French-fries, frozen			
(20 strips)			
Fried in oil	16	200	
Oven reheated	8	50	
Potatoes (½ cup)			
Scalloped	6	400	
Sweet, candied	3	50	8
Potato salad (½ cup)	10	650	2
Sauerkraut (½ cup)		800	
Tomato juice, canned (¾ cup)		650	

Vegetables (cont.)	Fat	Sodium	Sugars
Vegetables, canned with salt (½ cup)		250	
Vegetable soup, canned (1 cup)	2	800	

VENDING MACHINE FOODS

Values are based on approximate amounts per package or can. Sugar content is given only for desserts in this chart. Fat and sugar are listed by grams; sodium by milligrams.

Desserts	Fat	Sodium	Sugars
Brownie, frosted	5	50	11
Candy bar, milk chocolate (1.4 oz.)			
Plain	13	34	21
With almonds	15	34	20
With rice cereal	10	67	21
Candy bar, milk chocolate (2 oz.), with peanuts, caramel, and nougat	13	144	26
Cookie, chocolate chip (10 small cookies)	9	176	17
Donut, cake-type, plain	12	192	8

Main Dishes	Fat	Sodium	Sugars
Beef and macaroni (8-oz. can)	9	1,185	
Beef stew (7⅝-oz. can)	6	929	
Chili, chunky with beef (7½-oz. can)	6	820	
Soup, ready to serve			
Chicken noodle (7¼-oz. can)	2	765	
Vegetable (8-oz. can)	3	897	
Spaghetti and ground beef (7½-oz. can)	9	1,055	
Yogurt, low-fat (8-oz. carton)			
Flavored	3	149	
Fruit	2	133	

Snack Foods

	Fat	Sodium	Sugars
Crackers, cheese, with peanut butter (6)	12	540	
Corn chips (1-oz. pkg.)	9	233	
Peanuts, roasted in oil, salted (1-oz. pkg.)	14	122	
Potato chips (1-oz. pkg.)	10	132	
Raisins (½-oz. box)		2	
Sunflower seeds, hulled, roasted in oil, salted	16	171	

SANDWICH GUIDE

Use this guide to choose sandwich ingredients that are lower in fat, cholesterol, and sodium. Fat is listed in grams; sodium and cholesterol in milligrams.

Breads

	Fat	Sodium	Cholesterol
Croissant, 4½ × 4 × 1¾ in. thick (1)	12	452	13
Pita bread, 6½ in. in diameter	1	339	
Rye (2 slices)	2	350	
Whole wheat (2 slices)	2	360	

Sandwich Add-Ons

	Fat	Sodium	Cholesterol
Butter (1 tsp.)	4	39	10
Lettuce (1 leaf)		2	
Margarine (1 tsp.)	4	51	
Mayonnaise (1 tsp.)	4	26	3
Mayo-type light salad dressing (1 tsp.)		45	3
Mustard, prepared (1 tsp.)		63	
Relish, sweet pickle (1 tsp.)		36	
Tomato (two slices)		8	

Sandwich Fillings	*Fat*	*Sodium*	*Cholesterol*
Bologna (1 slice/1 oz.)	8	300	16
Cheese (1 slice/1 oz.)			
American, process	9	406	27
Swiss, natural	8	74	26
Ham, lean boiled (2 oz.)	3	815	27
Peanut butter (2 tbsp.)	16	150	
Roast beef (2 oz.)			
Deli	9	234	47
Home cooked, lean	4	37	46
Tuna salad, made with light tuna packed in oil, and mayo-type salad dressing (¼ cup)	5	206	7
Turkey, home-cooked, sliced (2 oz.)	3	40	43

INDEX